KUMBHAKA-

Science of prāṇāyāma

of

raghuvīra

Edited by

Dr. M. L. Gharote
Dr. Parimal Devnath

2005
The Lonavla Yoga Institute (India)
Lonavla—410401

First Edition, 2000,
Second Edition,
Lonavla, 2005

Printed by —
Capt. N. Dass (Rtd.),
XL Images,
411/1, Plot-11
J.C. Satish Agrawal Marg,
Dapodi,
Pune—411 012
India

Published by—
Dr. Manmath M. Gharote,
The Lonavla Yoga Institute (India).
A-7, Gulmohar Apartment,
Bhangarwadi,
Lonavla (India) 410 401

Rs. 295/-
$ 18
€ 15

ISBN 81-901176-5-3

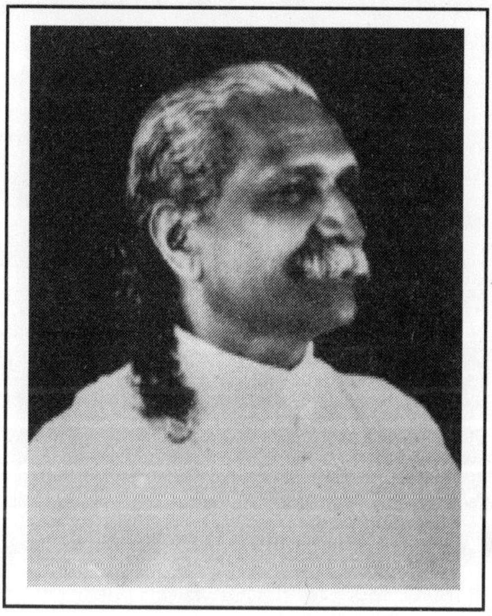

Dedicated
with
profound respects
to

Swami Kuvalayananda

who strongly emphasized
on the need of
literary research in Yoga

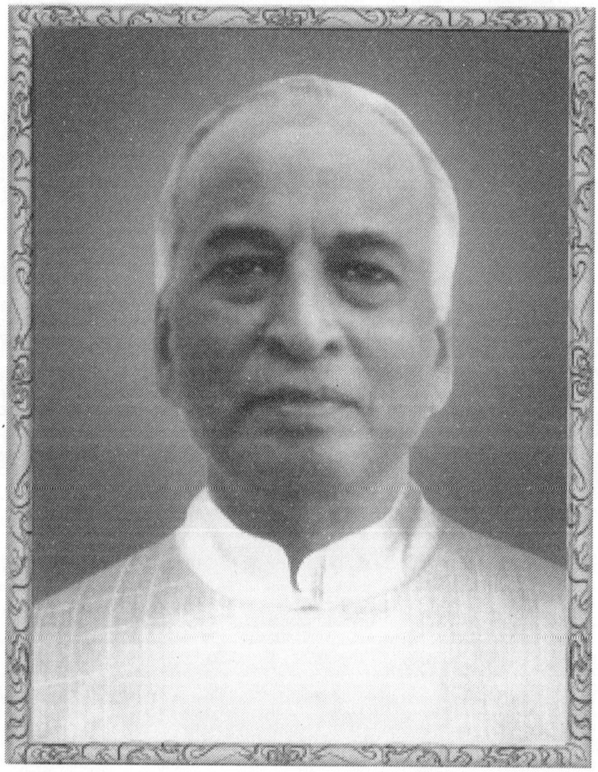

Dr. M. L. Gharote
21/05/1931 - 17/01/2005

Contents

List of Plates

The facsimile of the first page of the Manuscript No. B-6597 of *kumbhaka-paddhati* by *raghuvīra* deposited in the Asiatic Society Lib., Calcutta.

sahita-kumbhaka

kākacañcu-kumbhaka

Contents

Foreword

kumbhaka-paddhati (manual on *prāṇāyāma*) of *śrī raghuvīra*, edited by Dr. M. L. Gharote and Dr. Parimal Devnath is an interesting collection on the science of *prāṇāyāma*.

yoga-cūḍāmaṇi-upaniṣad mentions *prāṇāyāma vidyā* as *mahāvidyā* (great knowledge of learning), where the practitioner of *prāṇāyāma* experiences the union of himself with the Universal Spirit (*brahma*).

kumbhaka-paddhati explains fifty-seven types of *kumbhaka* with forty-seven stages.

God is one, but people call him by different names. Similarly, though the text explains fifty-seven types of *kumbhakas*, the readers should know that the principal *kumbhakas* are of these types namely, *antar-kumbhaka* (retention of breath after inhalation), *bāhya-kumbhaka* (retention of breath after exhalation), *kumbhaka* in-between interrupted *pūraka* and *recaka* and one that is both instinctive and intuitive (*kevala-kumbhaka*).

Actually, *prāṇāyāma* consists of four movements: *pūraka* (in-breath), *antar-kumbhaka* (retention after breath), *recaka* (out-breath) and *bāhya-kumbhaka* (retention of breath after the out-breath).

As different patterns of breathing and retention can be discovered while performing different types of *āsanas*, it is possible to adopt and adapt different types of breathing patterns and retention (*kumbhaka*), according to one' internal intellectual development and maturity. These adoptions and adaptations through the various permutations and combinations express the multiples of *kumbhakas*.

As *praṇava 'aum'* with the crescent and dot is the seed of all words, *pūraka* represents generation or creation of energy (G) *brahmā*, *antar-kumbhaka* represents organization of energy (O) *viṣṇu*, *recaka* releases that vitious air that destroys life (D) *maheśvara*, while *bāhya-kumbhaka* takes one to experience the changeless, eternal state of quietude.

prāṇāyāma is a great penance (*mahā tapas*). It is *nādānusandhāna*, one has to investigate, inquire and search (*śravaṇa, manana* and *nididhyāsana*). Lord *patañjali* puts this in simple words, *japa, artha* and *bhāvanā*.

We have all been bestowed with *pañca-bhautika-śarīra* consisting of earth, water, air and ether. They are the physical matters of the body. These five matters have their own infrastructures as *pañca tanmātrās*, namely, odour, taste, shape, touch and space. These *tanmātrās* are the chemistry and alchemy of the body. These are controlled by the cosmic life force (*viśva-prāṇa-śakti*). As nature (*prakṛti*) divides into various sections, this *viśva-prāṇa-śakti* transforms into *pañca vāyus* as *prāṇa, apāna, samāna, vyāna* and *udāna*. These five *vāyu's* locations have been explained in the text corresponding to the five elements and their corresponding five atomic powers. They also correspond to the five *cakras* namely, *mūlādhāra, svādhiṣṭhāna, maṇipūraka, anāhata* and *viśuddhi*. The other two *cakras, ājñā* and *sahasrāra* are beyond matter.

These *pañca-vāyus* churn, mix, mould and blend the *bhūtas* and *tanmātrās* to bring their essence (*rasa*) and *prāṇa śakti* (elixir of life).

We are endowed with *kāraṇa-śarīra* (causal body), *sūkṣma-śarīra* (subtle body) and *sthūla-śarīra* (gross body, also called *kārya-śarīra*).

These three bodies represent the *prajñā* (awareness) of self, consciousness and body (*asmitā, citta, deśa*) and *prāṇa* acts as the link in connecting these three bodies. For example, inhalation helps in expanding the self and consciousness progressively in delicate adjustment to touch the torso (*deśa*), whereas in exhalation, the sense and feel of the body and consciousness is gradually released to reach the self without any disturbance or collapse in the outer body. In *kumbhaka* equi-balance of *prāṇa* and *apāna* is learnt. This way *prāṇāyāma sādhānā* acts as a hub for the *sādhaka* to learn this connection with clarity.

In short, the secret of *prāṇāyāma* is the art of spacing the intelligence of the self, judiciously in the body (*deśa*), by *pūraka*. Uniting together the space in place is *antar-kumbhaka*. Releasing the breath delicately for the place to reach the inner space is *recaka*, bringing together the place with the interior space of the body is *bāhya-kumbhaka*. Hence, *prāṇāyāma* is not only a method of balancing the energy metabolism, but it also is an experiencing the state of composed consciousness (*samādhāna-citta*).

kumbhaka-paddhati cautions that, 'as one climbs from the lower steps to reach the top of the ladder, one has to progress in *kumbhaka*, carefully observing the rules and stages of *prāṇāyāma* to reach the higher stages of *yoga*' (KP-231-236). The effects of *kumbhaka* explained from 237 to 280 in this treatise are also found in the *vibhūti-pāda* of *patañjali* and *haṭhayoga* texts.

The notes given at the end of the book are a guide for *sādhakas*.

I feel that it is a valuable book for keen *prāṇāyāma sādhakas* and it is a well presented book to know and understand the richness of the science, art and philosophy of *prāṇāyāma*.

(Dr.) B. K. S. Iyengar

11th July 2000
Pune

PUBLISHER'S NOTE
First Edition

There are very few texts available which deal exclusively with the topic of *prāṇāyāma.* Besides the HP, GS, SS, YU, VS, BYS and a few works more, very little is known about the literature on *prāṇāyāma.* There are some compilations like YC, HR, HSC, HTK which elaborately deal with *prāṇāyāma* along with other topics. But they are still unpublished. We are working to prepare critical editions of these texts and will present to the readers in due course.

The text of *kumbhaka paddhati* in *sanskṛta* is uniquely devoted to the topic of *prāṇāyāma.* Although it seems to be quite recent a text of 19th century, it is based on the traditions and several *yoga* treatises and the information contained therein is not available elsewhere. *sundaradeva,* the author of HSC and HTK extensively quotes from *kumbhaka paddhati.*

The publication of the present work therefore must be considered as a welcome addition to the literature on *yogic* techniques.

The great defect in the *sanskṛta* writings on *yoga* is the frequent violation of the rules of grammar, metrics, etc. Repetition, ambiguity of expressions and incoherent presentation are also to be noticed. But these defects are insignificant in comparison with the high importance of the text from historical, practical, religious, philosophical and technical points of view. We hope, *yoga* teachers and students will be amply benefited from this text.

We are very grateful to Padmashri Yogacarya Dr. B K. S. Iyengar, who in spite of his busy schedule was kind enough to write Foreward to this book. This shows his sincere love for the cause of *yoga.*

We are grateful to Alicia Souto, Director, Centro de Eutony and Yogaterapia, Buenos Aires, Argentina, which is affiliated to the Lonavla Yoga Institute (India), for generously meeting the cost of publication.

Dr. Manmath M. Gharote

PUBLISHER'S NOTE
Second Edition

We are happy to present the Second Edition of *kumbhaka-paddhati* to the hands of the readers who highly appreciate our sincere effort to bring out the traditional texts on *yoga* critically edited in modern language. Due to good demand, the First Edition was exhausted and hence it has been out of print for some time. We therefore decided to bring out the second print of this text to meet the growing demand from the *yoga* enthusiasts.

In the present edition, we have arranged the text, transliteration, translation, critical notes, foot notes in this sequence to provide better readability. We hope that the discerning readers will benefit from this.

We express our sincere thanks to **Dr. V. K. Jha** and **Dr. Alicia Souto** who have minutely gone through the press copy of this book and suggested many valuable improvements.

Dr. Manmath M. Gharote

Scheme of Transliteration

Letters, their sounds and description of these sounds

Simple Vowels—

ॐ	om	like	o	in	home
अ	a	,,	a	,,	but
आ	ā	,,	a	,,	far
इ	i	,,	i	,,	pin
ई	ī	,,	ee	,,	feel
उ	u	,,	u	,,	fulsome
ऊ	ū	,,	oo	,,	wool
ऋ	ṛ	,,	r	,,	German

Dipthongs—

ए	e	,,	a	,,	fate
ऐ	ai	,,	ai	,,	aisle (but not drawled out)
ओ	o	,,	o	,,	over
औ	au	,,	ou	,,	ounce (but not drawled out)

Gutturals—

क	k	,,	k	,,	kill
ख	kh	,,	kh	,,	ink-horn
ग	g	,,	g	,,	girl
घ	gh	,,	gh	,,	longhouse
ङ	ṅ	,,	n	,,	king or ink

Palatals—

च	c	,,	ca	,,	church
छ	ch	,,	like the sound in Churchill		

ज	j	,,	j	in	join
झ	jh	,,	palatal 'z'	in	azure
ञ	ñ	,,	n	in	pinch

Cerebrals—

ट	ṭ	,,	t	,,	tub
ठ	ṭh	,,	th	,,	pot-house
ड	ḍ	,,	dh	,,	dog
ढ	ḍh	,,	dh	,,	mad-house
ण	ṇ	,,	n	,,	splinter or and

Dentals—-

त	t	,,	dental 't'	as in 'thin' or	like the French 'T'
थ	th	,,	th	in	thunder
द	d	,,	th	,,	then
ध	dh	,,	th	,,	this
न	n	,,	n	,,	no

Labials—-

प	p	,,	p	,,	paw
फ	ph	,,	ph	,,	top-heavy or gh in long
ब	b	,,	b	,,	balm
भ	bh	,,	bh	,,	hob-house
म	m	,,	m	,,	mat

Semi-vowels—

य	y	,,	y	,,	yawn
र	r	,,	r	,,	rub
ल	l	,,	l	,,	lo
व	v	,,	w	,,	wane

Spirants—-

श	ś	,,	sh	,,	ashes

ष	ṣ	,,	a strong lingual with rounded lips		
स	s	,,	s	,,	sun

Aspirate—-

ह	h	,,	h	,,	hum

Nasalised म् as in संयम (*saṃyama*) —ṃ
visarga———————————————ḥ

***

Abbreviations

BB-bālabodha
BPS-bṛhat-parāśara-saṃhitā
BrA-bṛhadāraṇyaka
BYS-bṛhadyogī-yājñyavalkya-smṛti
ChU-chāndogyopaniṣad
CS- caraka saṃhitā
DarU-darśanopaniṣad
DB-devī-bhāgavata
GP-gorakṣa-paddhati
GŚ-gorakṣa-śataka
GhS-gheraṇḍa-saṃhitā
HP-haṭhapradīpikā, Theosophical Publishing House.
HP(L)-haṭhapradīpikā (Lonavala Yoga Institute publication)
HP(K)- haṭhapradīpikā, Kaivalyadhama, Lonavla.
HR-haṭharatnāvalī (Lonavla Yoga Institute publication)
HSC- haṭha-saṅketa-candrikā(ms.)
HTK-haṭha-tatva-kaumudī (Lonavla Yoga Institute publication)
HMY-yogaśāstra of hemacandra
HY- haṭha-yoga
JP-joga-pradīpakā
KP-kumbhaka-paddhati
KūPu-kūrma-purāṇa
LPu-liṅga-purāṇa
MhB-mahābhārata
MPu-mārkaṇḍeya-purāṇa
PYS-pātañjala-yoga-sūtra
RY-rudryāmala
ŚanU-śāṇḍilyopaniṣad
SPu-saura-purāṇa
SD-svānubhava-dinakara
SŚe-siddhānta-śekhara
SN-ṣaṭ-cakra-nirūpaṇa

SPu-skanda-purāṇa
ŚS-śiva-saṃhitā
SSP-siddha-siddhānta-paddhati (Lonavla Yoga Institute publication)
SuS- suśruta saṃhitā
TBU- triśikha-brāhmaṇopaniṣad
TtA-taittirīya-āraṇyaka
VB-vyāsa-bhāṣya
VBh-vijñāna-bhairava
ViS-viṣṇu-saṃhitā
VāPu-vāyu-purāṇa
VS-vasiṣṭha-saṃhitā
YuB-yukta-bhavadeva
YC-yoga-cintāmaṇi
YM- Yoga Mīmāṃsā
YRah(N)-yogarahasya of nāthamuni
YSC-yoga-siddhānta-candrikā
YU-yogopaniṣads

***

Detailed Contents

(Numbers indicate verse numbers)

***

Fascimile of the first folio of the Ms. No.B-6597 of Asiatic Society Lib., Calcutta

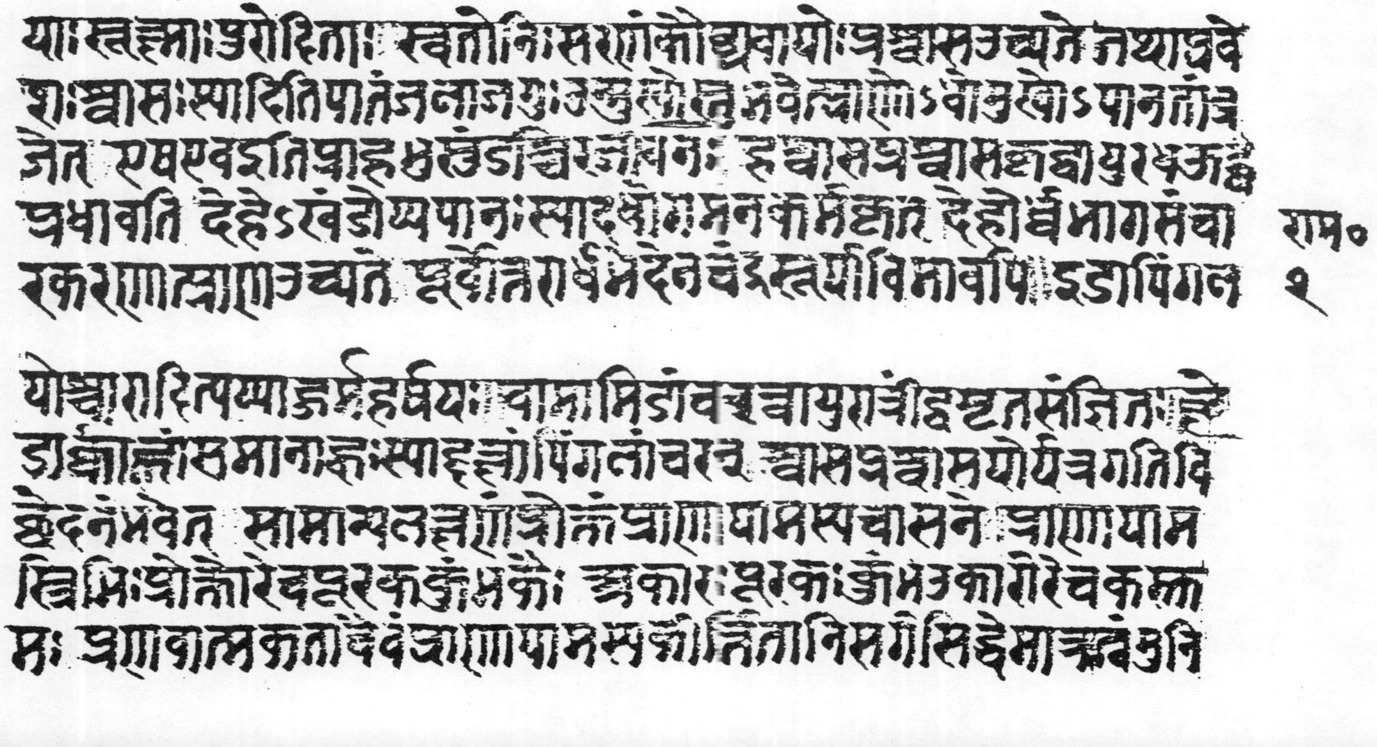

Introduction

The work of editing the present text of *kumbhaka paddhati* was started with the single manuscript available in the beginning. This manuscript is deposited in the Rajasthan Oriental Research Institute, Jodhpur the details of which are as follows—

Acc. No. 4577, *kumbhaka paddhati* by *raghuvīra.*

Size 24.0x11.3 cm., lines 10, letters 28, folio No. 21, status – complete, condition good, age 19th century.

This is indicated as 'J'.

As the work proceeded we found the quotations from *kumbhaka paddhati* in the works like HSC and HTK, both composed by *sundaradeva.* For comparison and variant readings, these quotations from *kumbhaka paddhati* were considered. When the text was almost completed, we came to know that another manuscript copy of *kumbhaka paddhati* is deposited in the Library of Asiatic Society, Kolkata, through our friend Dr. Dhanaraj Sharma, Prof. of Sanskrit Deptt., Punjab University, Chandigarh. He was kind enough to send us a Xerox copy of this manuscript for our study. We are grateful to him for his friendly gesture in the interest of *yoga*. The details of this manuscript are as follows—

Acc. No. viii.B.6597, Royal Asiatic Society of Bengal, Kolkata, *kumbhaka paddhati* by *raghuvīra audīcya*, I.M.499.

Size 22.5x9.3 cm., lines 5, letters 8-11, folio No. 31, status complete, condition good.

This is indicated as 'A'.

'J' manuscript is more complete. There are many verses missing in 'A' manuscript. However, 'A' manuscript has been used for determining important readings.

It is interesting to note that 'A' manuscript has been noted in the Aufrecht's Catalogus and in Catalogus Catalogrum. But the 'J' manuscript has not been included.

We find the 'J' manuscript important and therefore it is used as vulgate.

The author of *kumbhaka paddhati*

The author of *kumbhaka paddhati* is *raghuvīra*. He is also mentioned as *rāghava*, *raghupati* and *raghurāma*. He has given a brief account of himself in the beginning of the text from which we know that his father *śivarāma* hailed from a royal family and was residing in *kāśī* (Benares). He was a descendent of *kutsa gotra* (clan) and was an *udīcya brāhmaṇa*.

Kaivalyadhāma, Lonavla, has published a text called '*satkarma-saṃgraha*' edited by Dr. R. G. Harshe in 1970. In this text verse no. 148 states—

iti saṅkṣepataḥ proktaḥ karmaṇāṃ saṅgrahaḥ paraḥ ।
viduṣā raghuvīreṇa śrīman-nātha-prasādataḥ. ॥

This ascribes its authorship to *raghuvīra, rāghava* or *raghunātha*. In verse no. 149 there is a reference to *audīcya brāhmaṇa*—'*iti śrīmad-dvijodīcya-jñāti-rājakulābhidhāt*'. From these statements it is clear that *rāghava* or *raghuvīra* has also written the above text of *satkarma-saṃgrahaḥ*.

There are many similarities in his writings in both of these texts which may be mentioned below:

i) There are frequent references to the sources of *śiva* found in both the texts. Every now and then the author has expressed his indebtedness to *śiva* using several of *śiva's* synonyms.

ii) He calls himself an *audīcya brāhmaṇa* and descendent of a royal family.

iii) He calls his treatise on a particular subject as '*paddhati*' like '*karma-paddhati*' and '*kumbhaka-paddhati*'.

The text of *satkarma-saṃgraha* apparently seems to have been written by '*cidghanānandanātha*'—'*cidghanānandanātho'haṁ kurve satkarma-saṅgraham.*' It is possible that this name has been adopted by *raghuvīra* or *rāghava* prior to writing of the *'satkarma-saṅgraha'* as suggested by the editor of this text. He calls himself as the disciple of *gaganānanda-nātha*. *rāghava* seems to have written another text named *'miśraka'* having an admixture of *yoga* and medicine as the title indicates.

We come across quotations from KP in the works like *haṭhasaṅketa-candrikā* and *haṭha-tatva-kaumudī* authored by *sundaradeva*.

Both *raghuvīra* and *sundaradeva* were residing in *kāśī*. But it is not known whether they were contemporaries.

The title of the text

The title of the text given by the author is *kumbhaka paddhati*. He also refers to *kumbhamārga* or the path of *kumbhaka* originated from *śiva*. *kumbhaka paddhati* and *kumbhamārga* may be considered as synonyms.

What is *kumbhaka*?

The word *kumbhaka* is derived from the word *kumbha* meaning a water pot. Just as a water pot contains water, similarly, when the lungs hold the air, it is called *kumbhaka*. *yoga-yājñyavalkya* defines *kumbhaka* as *'sampūrṇa-kumbhavad-vāyor-dhāraṇaṃ kumbhako bhavet'*. *kumbha* is used for *kumbhaka* in many places in the present text. *kumbhaka* is also a synonym of *prāṇāyāma* and has been profusely used in the *paurāṇika* and *haṭhayogic* literature. In these texts, the technique of *prāṇāyāma* is described in three phases, namely, *pūraka, kumbhaka* and *recaka*. But in *prāṇāyāma* the phase of *kumbhaka* is most important and *pūraka* and *recaka* are only complementary and supplementary phases. Looking to the importance of the *kumbhaka* phase, it is considered as a synonym for *prāṇāyāma*. Thus the three phases of *prāṇāyāma*, namely, *pūraka, kumbhaka* and *recaka* are respectively the processes of filling the lungs with air, holding the air in the lungs and expelling the air from the lungs.

In the phase of *kumbhaka,* there is no movement of breath. Therefore, *smṛtis* define it as *niścala-śvāsaḥ.* It is a phase in the respiration technically described as *śvāsa-praśvāsa-gati-vicchedaḥ* (PYS-II.49).

Physiology of *kumbhaka*

kumbhaka may be physiologically described as Breath Holding. The term Breath Holding occurs frequently in the Sports literature. In many athletic events breath is held. The physiology of breath holding involves respiratory, circulatory and cardiac changes, all of which are important. Most obvious changes are increasing level of CO_2 and decreasing level of O_2 in the alveolar air. These changes reflect the changes in the level of respiratory gases in the blood. O_2 and CO_2 levels are involved in respiratory control, but CO_2 level is more important in holding the breath.

When the partial pressure of CO_2 in the alveolar air exceeds approximately 50mm.Hg., the stimulus to breathe is so strong that the breath can no longer be held. This is called Break Point at which breathing recommences.

Chemoreceptors are susceptible to chemical component of the blood. Due to accumulation of CO_2, the capacity to retain the breath is limited. According to Haldane .01 per cent change in CO_2 changes the action of the respiratory system.

In *kumbhaka* afferent impulses of Vagus start from the lungs and the efferent impulses of Vagus are sent back from Medulla oblongata. The afferent impulses enable us to keep the lungs in a particular stretched position and the efferent impulses help to slow down the heart.

When *bandhas* are applied during *kumbhaka*, the presso-receptors yield to internal and external pressure. Thus *jālandhara bandha* has its effect on carotid sinus and helps to maintain the stretching of the lungs and slowing down of the heart.

When *uḍḍiyāna* is applied, presso-receptors situated in the abdominal viscera come into play and help maintain the stretching of the lungs and slowing down of the heart.

Same effect is obtained by the application of *mūlabandha* which activates parasympathetic system resulting in slowing down of the heart.

All the three *bandhas* applied during *kumbhaka* have one and the same purpose.

By developing breath-holding time in *kumbhaka*, we may improve physiological function by slowing down the heart and metabolism in general. But the importance of *kumbhaka* lies in its psychological and spiritual effects. For this, control of emotions is very necessary. Respiratory activity is influenced by three factors, namely, metabolic, emotional and volitional. To take the advantage of volitional factor in *kumbhaka*, the other two disturbing factors must be controlled. For this Hypothalamus will have to be trained. It is by developing concentration that we can activate this. Therefore, mere holding of breath in *kumbhaka* is not enough, concentration is also necessary. *kumbhaka* without concentration will not help psychologically and spiritually. For the pacification of Hypothalamus and quietening it, practice of concentration is necessary. Therefore, during the practice of *kumbhaka*, various concentration points have been suggested. The very purpose of *kumbhaka* or *prāṇāyāma* as stated by *patañjali* is to create proper environment for concentration (*dhāraṇāsu ca yogyatā manasaḥ* PYS-II.53).

Practice of *kumbhaka* introduces high pressure, both in the central canal of the spinal cord and the ventricles of the brain. These pressures centrally stimulate the whole nervous system, which helps the human consciousness to be internalized and super conscious perceptions become possible.

Recently, Neuro-psychologists are taking considerable interest in breathing patterns and their effects on consciousness and the body functions. It has been observed that changes of electrical activity are directly correlated with the changes in the relative nostril dominance. It is also seen that greater integrated EEG value in one hemisphere correlates with the predominance of the contra-lateral nostril.

Dr. M. V. Rajapurkar has presented a hypothesis that, 'during *kumbhaka* the intra-nasal pressure increases, the conche helps form whirls, the intra-nasal temperature increases and the enclosed air absorbs more moisture from the vascular mucosa. All these changes stimulate the olfactory nerve endings in the superior meatus of the nose. The impulses are carried to the olfactory lobe which sits on the cribriform plate and is then transmitted via the olfactory nerves to the limbic lobe. The limbic lobe feeds into the hypothalamus and then into the cerebral cortex. This seems to be one of the mechanisms through which the results of *prāṇāyāma* on the psycho-spiritual level are attained.'

(Excerpt of the Paper presented in the 2nd International Conference on Yoga, Lonavla, 1988).

vāyu

With just a few exceptions, in *yoga* texts the words *vāyu, vāta, prāṇa, pavana, samīraṇa, anila, māruta, marut, śvasana, prabhañjana* are used indiscriminately as synonyms. This is confusing. It is necessary to consider the meaning of the word *vāyu* with reference to the context.

The various meanings of the word *vāyu* are—

i. Breath, i.e., the air that is breathed in and out,

ii. *prāṇa* which goes from *nābhimūla* (navel) to the head but can be carried to any part of the body and kept there for a shorter or longer time,

iii. Life, often used as *vāyavaḥ* in plural, signifying the many reflex activities,

iv. The *mahābhūta* (element) *vāyu*,

v. That region of the body where the *mahābhūta vāyu* is somehow said to reside,

vi. Nourishment, which reaches all the parts of the body—may be chiefly oxygen,

vii. Contraction of the muscles for performing an action,

viii. Ayurvedic *vāta-doṣa*—the wind which dries up things,

ix. The attitude of mind.

All these meanings of *vāyu* and its synonyms have to do with life, which is associated with movement. But *vāyu* and its synonyms signifying life and phenomena connected with life more than movement. Breathing, expiration, expired air, inspired air; all these are intimately connected with life. The ten vital reflexes are life. Nourishment maintains life. Contraction and expansation of muscles is a life activity. *vātadoṣa* is a defect in the processes of life. Nevertheless, always translating these words as life will not help us. We must see the distinctions between them and translate appropriately with reference to context.

prāṇa and *vāyu*

The word *prāṇa* is often used for *vāyu*. Different meanings of *prāṇa* found in the *yogic* literature are:

i. Vital force or the Principle of all the beings,

ii. Symbol of *brahmā*,

iii. A cosmic entity inhering both physical and material aspects of creation,

iv. A vibrating, pulsating or radiating type of energy,

v. Life process governing the activities of different living beings,

vi. Respiratory air,

vii. The air sent out during exhalation or a stimulus for exhalation,

viii. Respiratory impulse causing inhalation or exhalation,

ix. Nervous impulse or sensation passing through different parts of the body,

x. Ten vital reflexes forming the life function related to conscious and unconscious activity of the body conditioned by Time and Space.

prāṇa and *vāyu* are the terms which have been used interchangeably in the *kumbhaka paddhati.*

The *prāṇādi-vāyus* are usually enumerated as ten. They are *prāṇa*, *apāna*, *samāna*, *udāna*, *vyāna*, *nāga*, *kūrma*, *kṛkara*, *devadatta* and *dhanañjaya*. Of these ten, the first five are principal and of these five also again *prāṇa* and *apāna* are the most important (ŚS-III.6). These *prāṇādi-vāyus* constitute what is called life-process or *jīvana* as *vyāsa* calls it (VB-III.39).

As this process is promoted by *prāṇādi-vāyus* (i.e. autonomic functions) and carried on in the different parts of the body, writers on *yoga* differentiate the *prāṇādi-vāyus* with reference to the different locations of these autonomic functions.

The locations, sphere of activity and the color of the *prāṇādi-vāyus* is given in the following table:

Description of *prāṇādi-vāyus*

Name		Location	Color
Activity 1. ***prāṇa***	From nose and mouth to chest	Green (YuB, HY), dull red (ViS)	Respiration
2. ***apāna***	From abdomen to soles of feet	Black (YuB, HY), red (ViS)	Excretion of urine, faeces and foetus
3. ***samāna***	From chest to the abdomen	White (YuB, HY), transparent (ViS)	Even distribution of essence of food - in various parts of the body
4. ***udāna***	From nose and mouth to the head	Red, (YuB, HY) white (ViS)	Sending up secretions or juices
5. ***vyāna***	Pervades the whole body	Rainbow (YuB, HY) bright yellow (ViS)	Various movements of the body

The functions of the five *nāgādi* minor *vāyus* are mentioned in ŚS-III.8 as follows: *nāga* causes eructation, *kūrma* causes the eyes to open, *kṛkara* causes hunger and thirst, *devadatta* causes yawning and *dhanañjaya* causes hiccup.

The SSP-I.69 has a different description about the functioning of the ten *vāyus*. It is said that:

(i) exhalation and inhalation are both caused by *prāṇa-vāyu*,

(ii) *apāna* is mainly responsible for the three phases of *prāṇāyāma*, viz. *recaka, kumbhaka* and *pūraka*. It appears that according to *gorakṣa, prāṇāyāma* is possible mainly by the action of *apāna*,

(iii) *samāna* is appetizer and digestive,

(iv) *vyāna* removes disorders in the *nāḍīs*,

(v) *udāna* helps swallowing or vomiting and talking,

(vi) *nāga* helps movements,

(vii) *kūrma* shakes the body and causes twinkling of the eyes,

(viii) *kṛkara* causes eructation and hunger,

(ix) *devadatta* causes yawning and

(x) *dhanañjaya* causes *nāda-ghoṣa* (sound).

Thus we find that in *yogic* literature the word *prāṇa* has a wide range of application, viz., from mere breath to a subtle cosmic principle.

To sum up, *prāṇa* means:

(i) Breath,

(ii) Respiratory impulse which causes inhalation and exhalation,

(iii) Nervous impulse or sensation passing through the different parts of the body,

(iv) Life process characterized by autonomic nervous functions in the various parts of the body,

(v) A cosmic entity, an evolute from *avyakta* pervading or inhering both the physical and a material aspects of creation.

It is also possible to think of the two aspects of *prāṇā*—static and dynamic—denoted by the words *prāṇā-śakti* (*prāṇā* as a power) and *prāṇa-vāyu* (*prāṇa* as a current) respectively.

Therapeutic aspects of breathing

Today *yoga* has become popular throughout the world due to its therapeutical aspect, especially to deal with psychosomatic problems caused by stressful situations.

It has been accepted that emotions affect breathing process. It is becoming equally clear that breathing patterns affect emotionality. Scientists have verified that the slightest change in respiration induces changes in the rest of the autonomic nervous system and that physiological reaction is an essential component in emotionality. Inadequate respiration produces anxiety irritability and tension. Inability to breathe normally is the main obstacle to the recovery of emotional health. Breathing forms a bridge between conscious and the unconscious. Our breathing pattern expresses our inner situation. Through *prāṇāyāmic* techniques of *yoga* one learns to consciously alter one's breathing and thus one's emotional state. Many *yogic* breathing techniques lead one towards deep relaxation. For example, one can attain a calm and alert state through smooth and even diaphragmatic breathing. Through conscious alteration of the breathing pattern one can modify autonomic arousal and modulate subsequent level of emotionality. A few schools of modern psychology and physiotherapy like Reichian Therapy, Bioenergetic Therapy utilize this concept.

As mentioned above, particular breathing irregularities are associated with specific emotional and psychosomatic disorders. These could be overcome by diaphragmatic breathing and an altered ratio of inhalation and exhalation. Breathing and thinking are interrelated and they influence one another. In *yoga*, breath has been used as a tool for regulating all of one's emotional and mental states and even the way in which one behaves.

Rationale of *kumbhaka*

When breath is active mind is also active. When breath is held, mind becomes inactive. Thus a *yogī* attains stability. Therefore, it should be practised (HP-II.2, IV.21,23-24).

Breath is the intermediary between body and mind. By developing breath awareness one develops awareness of the mind. Mindfulness for breathing leads on its own to the transcendence of ego, desires and suffering.

Breath, posture and thinking are interrelated. Unless the body is stable, mind cannot be steady. When the body is stable, the respiratory rate also comes down, subsequently reducing the thoughts.

According to PYS-II.52-53, the purpose of *kumbhaka* or *prāṇāyāma* is twofold —

(i) Reducing the domination of egoistic thoughts preventing proper knowledge of Reality (*prakāśāvaraṇa-kṣaya*) and,

(ii) Qualifying the mind for concentration (*dhāraṇāsu ca yogyatā manasaḥ*).

It brings stabilization of *prāṇic* currents contributing to the healthy mind and body and arousal of *kuṇḍalinī* force.

Traditions of *kumbhaka*

The author states in the introduction that he has composed the *kumbhaka paddhati* based on the traditions and in consideration of the essence of several texts on *yoga*. The tradition mainly referred to by him is *śiva* Himself. His expression '*kumbhamārgaṃ śivoditaṃ*' indicates the fact clearly. While referring to various techniques of *kumbhaka* he mentions traditions of such authorities like *patañjali*, *bhuśuṇḍa*, *kṛṣṇa-dvaipāyana*, *devala*, *dvikarāja*, *gonardīya*, *dattātreya*, *mārkaṇḍeya* and *aśvinī-kumāra* and other *ṛṣis* and *munis* along with the various commentators. For *śiva*, several synonyms have been used while describing different techniques attributed to *śiva*. They are: *bhālanetra*, *śaṅkara*, *caṇḍātmaja, candramauli, svayaṃbhū, śrīkṛttivāsa, druhiṇa, pārvatīpati, parameśvara, ādinātha, śaṃbhu, trinetra, mṛḍa, sadāśiva, dhūrjaṭi, viśvanātha, kapardi, tripurāntaka.* Thus it will be found that the main tradition of *kumbhaka* comes from *śiva.*

With the help of different traditions of *kumbhaka* we could trace the gross evolution of *kumbhaka.* This evolution could be divided broadly in five stages as described by Swāmī Kuvalayānanda in his article on the 'Evolution of Prāṇāyāma' (YM-VI.I:55-59). These stages could be assigned to different periods as follows:

First stage:— Religioius *sūtra* period,

In this stage, *kumbhaka* is only a part of some religious ceremony. There is no mention of *pūraka* and *recaka.*

Second stage:— *smṛti* period,

kumbhaka is accompanied with *gāyatrī, vyāhṛti, praṇava* and *śiras* or meditation on *brahmā, viṣṇu* and *maheśa* as obligatory. This attained an independent position as religious act; although it still occupied subordinate position in religious ceremonies.

Third stage:— *paurāṇic* period,

kumbhaka attained an independent position and not attached to any ritual. It was a part of spiritual practices to be accompanied by mental recitation of *praṇava* or *om.* Time units for *pūraka, kumbhaka* and *recaka* were introduced.

Fourth stage:— *yogasūtra* period,

kumbhaka or *prāṇāyāma* became an independent part of the psycho-physiological science. Credit goes to *patañjali* who discarded even the recitation of *praṇava* from the technique. *patañjali* does not use the word *kumbhaka.* His synonymous word is *prāṇāyāma* of which four varieties have been mentioned.

Fifth stage:— *haṭhayoga* period,

haṭhayoga emphasizes on internal *kumbhaka* and divides the technique in eight varieties based on the technique of *recaka* and *pūraka*. Every variety requires time units for *pūraka*, *kumbhaka* and *recaka* as 1:4:2 and is accompanied by *mūlabandha*, *jālandhara bandha* and *uḍḍiyāna bandha*. Different physiological results are attributed to different types of *kumbhaka*, which are expressed in Ayurvedic terms.

nāḍīśuddhi

nāḍīśuddhi or purification of *nāḍīs* (channels) is an important concept in *yoga*. It is maintained that unless the *nāḍīs* are purified further progress in *prāṇāyāma* and meditation is not possible. The purpose of all the preliminary processes of *bahiraṅga-yoga* is to attain *nāḍīśuddhi*.

Earliest reference to the *nāḍīs* is found in two of the oldest *upaniṣads*, namely, *chāndogya* and *bṛhadāraṇyaka*, according to which *nāḍīs* are as minute as a hair split a thousand times and are filled with humours of different colours. From the point of modern language, we may call them nerves along which motor and sensory impulses travel in the form of *vāyus* and perform different physical and mental functions. These could also be blood vessels. They are a part of the gross body, which is made of the five elements. They do not belong to the subtler or *sūkṣma* world. For elaborate discussion on the *nāḍīs*, see note on *gorakṣa-śataka* edited by Swāmī Kuvalayānanda and S. A. Shukla.

While giving rationale of *nāḍīśuddhi*, HP and GŚ state, "If the *nāḍīs* are full of impurities, *māruta (prāṇa)* does not travel along the middle path. How can then one attain the state of *unmanī (samādhi)* ? How can one succeed in attaining one's aim in *yoga*?"

Out of all the *nāḍīs*, a great importance is given to *suṣumnā nāḍī*. Therefore, ultimately *nāḍīśuddhi* refers to the stimulation of the *suṣumnā nāḍī*. All the processes of *nāḍīśuddhi* including *prāṇāyāma* are meant for removing the impurities of *suṣumnā*.

According to GhS-V.36), purification of *nāḍīs* is of two kinds: *samanu* and *nirmanu*. *samanu nāḍīśuddhi* is done with the help of *bījamantras*, while *nirmanu nāḍīśuddhi* is done by *ṣaṭkarmas* like *dhauti*, *basti* etc.

Different authorities emphasize on different techniques for *nāḍīśuddhi* right from *yamas* and *niyamas* (HSC, VS-I.81), *āsanas* (HP-I.39, RY-24-39), *prāṇāyāma* (HP-II.38) and food intake. According to some authorities, *prāṇāyāma* alone removes all impurities of the body.

The effects of *nāḍīśuddhi* have been described in HP-II.19 and KP-119-120 as follows—

"When the *nāḍīs* get purified, there appear external signs like slimness of the body and lustre. One is able to retain breath with ease, gastric fire is increased, there is an experience of internally aroused sound and good health is secured."

Physiologically these results may be expressed as follows—

i) Impulses are properly transmitted through the nerves which produce normal functions in a state of health.

ii) Any sort of pressure upon any part of the nervous system affects the efficiency of the nervous system, exaggerating or diminishing its capacity for transmitting impulses.

iii) Pressure can be caused by substances adjacent to the nerves, by irritation of the sensory nerves, by toxins which can irritate sensory nerves, including muscular contractions with a resultant pulling of the bone out of its current positions. Such pressures are removed as a result of *nāḍīśuddhi*.

As stated earlier, *prāṇāyāma* has been used as a potential technique of *nāḍīśuddhi*. In KP-114-120, three kinds of technique are given along with different visualizations as follows—

i) One should inhale through one nostril and after holding the breath to the capacity, exhale through the other nostril while contemplating on *haṃsa*. Then inhale through the nostril through which one has exhaled and repeat the process.

ii) Inhale through the right nostril, hold the breath to the capacity and concentrate in the navel on the orb of the mid-day sun of the summer.

iii) Inhale through the left nostril, hold the breath and while holding the breath visualize oozing of the nectar from the moon of the autumn night, situated in the lotus of thousand petals in the head.

VS, however, makes a difference between *nāḍīśuddhi* and *prāṇāyāma* and emphasizes on *nāḍīśuddhi* before taking to the practice of *prāṇāyāma*. According to it, purification of the *nāḍīs* is a prerequisite of *prāṇyāma* and not the result of *prāṇāyāma*. The technique of *nāḍīśodhana* given is in the form of *pūraka* and *recaka*. One should first exhale through one nostril followed by inhalation through the same nostril. Then one should exhale through the other nostril. Through this nostril he should perform inhalation followed by exhalation through the other. *vasiṣtha* calls this process as *nāḍī-śodhana*. SŚe describes seven (?) kinds of *nāḍī-śuddhi* (though this text mentions of seven varieties of *nāḍī-śuddhi*, but actually it describes only six). These are as follows:

i) Exhale through the free nostril. Then inhale through one nostril and exhale through the other after retention of breath. Repeat this process which is called *nāḍī-śuddhi* narrated by *brahmā*.

ii) Inhale through *iḍā nāḍī* and after holding the breath exhale through the other *nāḍī (piṅgalā)*. This is *raudrī nāḍī-śuddhi*.

iii) Inhale through one nostril and exhale through the other. (Practise it for sixteen times with three or four sittings per day for a period of four months). This is *vaiṣṇavī nāḍī-suddhi*.

iv) Inhale through both the nostrils and exhale through both.

v) Inhale through one nostril and exhale through both.

vi) Inhale through *iḍā*, the left nostril and after holding the breath, judiciously exhale through the other nostril.

TBU-I.31-33 provides a different interpretation of *prāṇāyāma*. According to this text, when one considers everything like *citta* etc. as *brahma* and controls all the modifications (of the mind) it is called *prāṇāyāma*.

recaka means overcoming of all the worldly attachments.

The attitude that 'I-am-*brahma*' is called *pūraka* and to maintain such a state is *kumbhaka*.

pratyāhāra

The usual meaning of *pratyāhāra* as withdrawing sense organs from the sense objects as described by PYS-II.54 or in GS-V.2-7, is not intended in KP. According to KP, withdrawing *prāṇa* from all the 18 vital points one after another in sequence is *pratyāhāra*. It is called *kumbhaka* by the *ṛṣiṣ*. It is done in a sequential and in reverse order during *kumbhaka*.

Four types of *pratyāhāra* have been mentioned in VS. They are described as follows :

i) Withdrawal of sense organs, which are indulged naturally in the sense objects.

ii) Everything that one sees should be seen as Self within the Self.

iii) Performance of the obligatory duties, mentally within the self and without any external aids is also *pratyāhāra.*

iv) Holding the *prāṇa* successively at the eighteen vital points after withdrawing from the previous points is *pratyāhāra.*

Along with the above four types of *pratyāhāra,* SanU-I.8 mentions fifth type of *pratyāhāra* in the form of renouncing the results of the daily obligatory duties. DarU-VII also endorses the same view.

In KP the term *pratyāhāra* has been used synonymously for *kumbhaka.* Thus, inhaling and holding the *prāṇa* from the heart upward upto the top of the head is called *uttara,* while holding it from top of the head downward upto the heart is called *adhara* according to the *munis.*

devala mentions seven types of *kumbhaka* out of which *pratyāhāra* is one.

The classification of *pūraka, recaka* and *kumbhaka* is presented below :-

Classification of *pūraka, recaka* and *kumbhaka*

Classification of *pūraka*

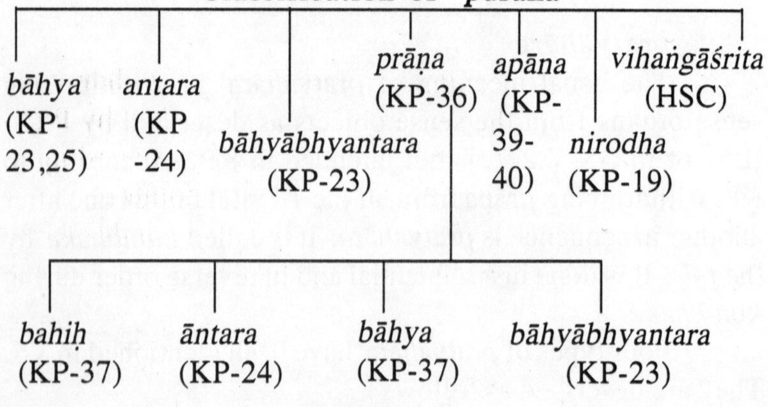

pūrakas—

A brief description of the *pūrakas* is presented below—

1. ***bāhyapūraka*** (KP-23,35)—The breath moving into the nose from a distance of twelve digits (nine inches) is called *bāhyapūraka*.

2. ***antara-pūraka*** (KP-24)—When inhaled air enters the opening of *suṣumnā* it is called *antara-pūraka*.

3. ***bāhyābhyantara-pūraka*** (KP-23)—When the air moves in the chest it is called *bāhyābhyantara-pūraka*.

4. ***bāhya-prāṇa-pūrakas*** (KP-35-37)—

a) When the external *vāyu* enters the lungs to its limit, it is *bāhya-prāṇa-pūraka* (KP-36).

b) According to *kāka*, when the air comes out of the body and moves up to twelve digits (nine inches) it is *bāhya-prāṇa-pūraka* or *bahiḥ-prāṇa-pūraka* (KP-37).

c) *prāṇa* which has a natural tendency to move upwards from the chest cavity, when controlled is called *bāhya-pūraka* (KP-35).

5. ***apāna-pūraka*** (KP-39-40)—

i) When *vāyu* moves into the nose from twelve digits outside, it is *āntara-apāna-pūraka* (KP-39).

ii) When *prāṇa* enters into the end of the nose from outside, it is *apāna-pūraka* (KP-40).

iii) When the air enters the chest from the tip of the nose it is also called *apāna-pūraka* (KP-40).

6. ***nirodha-pūraka*** (KP-19)—When the external air is inhaled either through the nose or the mouth it is *nirodha-pūraka*.

7. ***vihaṅgāśrita*** (HSC)—The air named *agni* while moving inside, supports the body of a *yogī*. When managed, it offers illumination. This is called *vihaṅgāśrita*. The description is not clear.

Classification of *recaka*

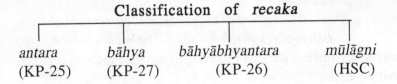

antara (KP-25)	*bāhya* (KP-27)	*bāhyābhyantara* (KP-26)	*mūlāgni* (HSC)

***recaka*—**

A brief description of *recakas* follows—

1. ***antara-recaka*** (KP-25)— When *vāyu* goes out of the opening of *suṣumnā* it is *antara-recaka.*

2. ***bāhya-recaka*** (KP-27)—When *prāṇa* moves in the space up to twelve digits (nine inches) from the tip of the nose, it is *bāhya-recaka.*

3. ***bāhyābhyantara-recaka*** (KP-26)—When the air moves up to the end of the nostrils from the thoracic cavity, it is *bāhyābhyantara-recaka.*

4. ***mūlāgni-recaka*** (HSC)—*agni* (fire) of *recaka* dries up the host of *pitta* (bile) and streamlines the digestion and also brings control on *pṛthivī* element. The technique is not very clear.

Classification of *kumbhaka*

(internal)	(external)	*(kevala)*
antaḥ ku. (KP-28)	*bahiḥ ku.* (KP-31)	*stambha-vṛtti* (PYS-II.50)
bāhyābhyantara (KP-29)	*recita ku.* (KP-31, *devala*)	*kevala* (HP(L)-IV.33,64-66)
pūrita ku. (KP-30, *devala*)	*prāṇa ku.* (KP-34)	*saṅghaṭṭa-karaṇa* (SSP-II.35)
apāna ku. (KP-34)	*sarva-śūnyaka* (KP-33)	*śānta* (*devala*)
ābhyantara-vṛtti (PYS-II.50-51)	*bāhya-vṛtti* (PYS-II.50-51)	*sama* (*devala*)
pūraka ku. (HSC)	*śūnyaka* (Sau.P)	

***kumbhaka*—**

A brief description of three types of *kumbhaka* is as follows—

1. **Internal *kumbhaka*—**

i) ***antaḥ-kumbhaka*** (KP-28)—When *prāṇa* is retained in *suṣumnā* without mental distraction, it is *antaḥ-kumbhaka*.

ii) ***bāhyābhyantara-kumbhaka*** (KP-29)— When inhaled air is retained in the chest cavity without reference to *suṣumnā* it is *bāhyābhyantara-kumbhaka*.

iii) ***pūrita-kumbhaka*** (KP-30)—*bāhyābhyantara-kumbhaka* is also called *pūrita-kumbhaka*.

iv) ***apāna-kumbhaka*** (KP-34)— According to *dvikarāja*, with inhaled air it is *apāna-kumbhaka*.

v) ***ābhyantara-vṛtti*** (PYS-II.50-51)—Breath is held internally.

vi) ***pūraka-kumbhaka*** (HSC)—Slowly inhale the external air and fill up the cavity. Move it to all the parts of the body. When the whole body is filled with air, carefully retain it. This is to be practised for one year.

2. **External *kumbhaka*—**

i) ***bahiḥ-kumbhaka*** (KP-31)—When air is exhaled slowly and breath is held outside it is *bahiḥ-kumbhaka*.

ii) ***recita-kumbhaka*** (KP-31)—*bahiḥ-kumbhaka* is also called *recita-kumbhaka*.

iii) ***prāṇa-kumbhaka*** (KP-34)—With exhaled air it is *prāṇa-kumbhaka*.

iv) ***sarva-śūnyaka*** (KP-33)—When the air is exhaled through the right nostril while mentally repeating *gāyatrī* along with *praṇava, vyāhṛti* and *śiras* and the breath is held outside, while contemplating on the internal void, it is *sarva-śūnyaka*.

v) ***bāhyavṛtti*** (PYS-II.50-51)—Suspension of external breath.

vi) **śūnyaka** (Sau.P)—After exhalation hold the breath outside without inhaling the air. Contemplate on the moon inside and absorb the nectar oozing form it.

3. ***kevala-kumbhaka*—**

stambhavṛtti (PYS-II.50)—When the breath is held without prior inhalation or exhalation it is called *stambhavṛtti*. This is variously known as *kevala-kumbhaka* (HP(L)-IV.33,64-66), *saṃghaṭṭa-karaṇa* (SSP-II.35), *śānta* and *sama (devala).*

[With one-pointed awareness of *antaḥ-kumbhaka* and *bahiḥ-kumbhaka* the mind becomes introverted and the activity of both *prāṇa* and *apāna* ceases and *suṣumnā* opens up (VBh-25).

By means of continuous practice of *kumbhaka*, physical and mental tranquility is experienced. The difference between *prāṇa* and *apāna* disappears. That is why *prāṇa-śakti* is known as *śānta* (VBh-27).

By the fusion (*saṃghaṭṭa-karaṇa*) of *prāṇa* and *apāna* there arises finally a condition in which there is complete cessation of breath whether inside or outside. By meditating over this condition, the *yogī* comes across the intuitive experience of equality (*samatva-vijñāna-samudgama*) (VBh-64)].

According to *devala* (quoted by *śivānanda* in *yogacintāmaṇi* ms. Folio no. 90), there are 7 varieties of *kumbhaka* which are narrated below—

i) **recita-kumbhaka**— Same as KP-31.

ii) **pūrita-kumbhaka**—Same as KP-30.

iii) **uttara-kumbhaka**—Holding of *prāṇa* above in the chest cavity followed by inhalation is *uttara-kumbhaka.*

iv) **adhara-kumbhaka**—Holding of *prāṇa* followed by inhalation in the lower cavity is *adhara-kumbhaka.*

v) **sama-kumbhaka**—Mental holding of *prāṇa* is *sama-kumbhaka.*

vi) ***pratyāhāra-kumbhaka***—Retention of *prāṇā* in-between the following points such as soles of the feet, generative organ, navel, chest, heart, throat, uvula, centre of the eyebrows, forehead and *brahmarandhra* is *pratyāhāra-kumbhaka.*

vii) ***śānta***— When *prāṇa* is retained followed by exhalation in the above mentioned points starting from the head up to chest it is *śānta-kumbhaka.*

Classification of *kumbhaka*

sahita

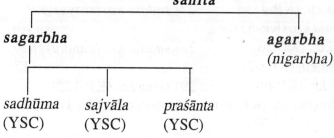

- ***sagarbha***
  - *sadhūma* (YSC)
  - *sajvāla* (YSC)
  - *praśānta* (YSC)
- ***agarbha*** *(nigarbha)*

sagarbha-kumbhaka—

According to YSC-II.51 *sagarbha-kumbhaka* has three varieties, namely, *sadhūmaka, sajvāla* and *praśānta* which are in short narrated below—

i) ***sadhūmaka***—Meditation on *mantra (om)* along with its three syllables is *sadhūmaka.*

ii) ***sajvāla***—Meditation on *mantra (om)* along with its syllables and meaning and their presiding deities is *sajvāla.*

iii) ***praśānta***—Meditation on attributeless represented by the *mantra (om)* along with *yoganāḍī (suṣumnā)* is *praśānta.*

Classification of *kumbhaka*

sahita

sagarbha — ***agarbha*** *(nigarbha)*

1) *antaḥ-ku.* (KP-28)
2) *bahiḥ-ku.* (KP-31)
3) *cāndra ku.* (KP-41)
4) *ūrdhvaja ku.* (KP-55)
5) *mṛga ku.* (KP-56)
6) *samāna ku.* (KP-62)
7) *vyāna ku.* (KP-66)
8) *kṛtti-śreṣṭha ku.* (KP-69)
9) *prakṛti ku.* (KP-70)
10) *nāga ku.* (KP-78)
11) *kūrma ku.* (KP-79)
12) *kṛkara-ku.* (KP-80)
13) *sahita-ku.* (KP-85)
14) *agni-ṣoma ku.* (KP-87)
15) *sama-ku.* (KP-99)
16) *śānta-ku.* (KP-90)
17) *karṣaka ku.* (KP-100)
18) *utkarṣaka ku.* (KP-101)
19) *apakarṣaka ku.* (KP-102)
20) *sahaja ku.* (KP-104)
21) *dakṣiṇāvarta cakra ku.* (KP-106)
22) *vāmāvarta cakra ku.* (KP-106)
23) *dakṣiṇāvarta śaṅkha ku.* (KP-106)
24) *vāmāvarta śaṅkha ku.* (KP-106)
25) *gadā ku.* (KP-112)
26) *nāḍīśuddhi-ku.* (KP-115)
27) *śuddhi ku. (sūrya)* (KP-116)
28) *śuddhi ku. (candra)* (KP-117)
29) *tatva ku.* (KP-122)
30) *sūrya-bhedana ku.* (KP-127)
31) *candra-bhedana ku.* (KP-128)
32) *ujjāyī ku.* (KP-132)
33) *kumbha-rāja* (KP-134)
34) *śitalī ku.* (KP-136)
35) *sītkārī ku.* (KP-136-140)
36) *kāka-cañcu ku.* (KP-141,148)
37) *śītalī-kāka-cañcu ku* (KP-143)
38) *mātrā ku.* (KP-153, 201-203)
39) *bhūta-śuddhi-ku.* (KP-157)
40) *bhastrikā-ku.* (KP-164-168)
41) *antaraṅga ku.* (KP-168)
42) *bhrāmarī ku.* (KP-169)

continued....

--*continued*

43) *mūrcchanā ku.* (KP-170)
44) *plāvinī ku.* (KP-171)
45) *svaṅga śṛṅkhalā ku.* (KP-178)
46) *kumbhāntara-śṛṅkhalā ku.* (KP-183)
47) *jīvacāla ku.* (KP-185)
48) *ṣaḍaṅga ku.* (KP-187)
49) *kamala ku.* (KP-189)
50) *kumuda ku.* (KP-190)
51) *krama-netra ku.* (KP-191)
52) *netra ku.* (KP-191)
53) *trinetra ku.* (KP-192)
54) *triśūla ku.* (KP-193)
55) *eka-meru ku.* (KP-206)
56) *dvi-meru ku.* (KP-207)
57) *tri-meru ku.* (KP-207)
58) *ghaṭī-bandha ku.* (KP-211)
59) *kālāgni ku.* (HSC)
60) *nāda ku.* or *lambā-guru-prānāyāma* (HSC)
61) *utkrānti prāṇāyāma* (HTK ch.53)
62) *vāma-gati & vartma-gati ku.* (HSC, HTK-X.28)
63) *bhujaṅgī-karaṇa* (HR-II.32,HY)
64) *bhuyaṅgama* (JP-V.487-490)
65) *trāṭaka ku.* (JP-V.491-493)
66) *kaṇṭhī-vetālī ku.* (JP-V.494-498)
67) *bhoralikā-ku.* (JP-V.477-481)
68) *kevalī-ku.* (GŚ)
69) *śūnyaka kumbhaka* (SauP-XII. 22-24)
70) *kevala kumbhaka*

kumbhakas

A brief description of these *kumbhakas* is as follows :

1. **ābhyantara kumbhaka** or **antaḥ-ku.** (KP-28) (internal retention of breath)

When breath is held inside after inhalation, it is the general nature of *ābhyantara kumbhaka*. It is variously named as *pūrita, pūraka, apāna, antaḥ* and *bāhyābhyantara kumbhaka*.

When *prāṇa* is retained in *suṣumṇā nāḍī* it is called *antaḥ kumbhaka*.

2. ***bāhya kumbhaka*** or ***bahiḥ-ku.*** (KP-31) (external retention of breath)

When breath is held outside after exhalation, it is called *bāhya kumbhaka, recita, bahiḥ, prāṇa kumbhaka, śūnyaka* and *sarva-śūnyaka.*

3. ***cāndra kumbhaka*** (KP-41)

After inhalation one holds the breath simultaneously applying *mūla-bandha* to stimulate *apāna vāyu.* This is *cāndra-kumbhaka* which brings control of *prāṇa* and *apāna.*

4. ***ūrdhvaja kumbhaka*** (KP-55)

After holding the breath when one practises *recaka*, one should visualize the moon at the base of the spine and concentrate from place to place going upwards along the spine.

5. ***mṛga kumbhaka*** (KP-56)

When *apāna* is held in the back of the hip region continuously, it is known as *mṛga kumbhaka.* This requires adoption of *mūla-bandha* and concentration in that region.

6. ***samāna kumbhaka*** (KP-62)

When *samāna vāyu* is held at the navel region with concentration, it is *samāna kumbhaka.* It helps in attaining *uḍḍīyāna,* increasing gastric fire, control of hunger and thirst, quick healing of wounds and fractures.

7. ***vyāna kumbhaka*** (KP-66)

Inhale deeply and hold the breath by contracting the whole body with subtle concentration. It gives protection from weapons, water and poisons, removes diseases and provides immunity from heat and cold.

8. ***kṛtti-śreṣṭha kumbhaka*** (KP-69)

The technique consists of holding the breath with progressive concentration in the throat, palate, mid-brow, top of the head and maintaining it there.

9. ***prakṛti kumbhaka*** (KP-70)

Sucking the air in with a loud sound and holding the breath is known as *prakṛti kumbhaka*.

10. ***nāga kumbhaka*** (KP-78)

One should swallow the air into the throat like taking a morsel of rice. Then retain the breath to the capacity with firm *jālandhara bandha* and expel the air from the throat. This is the technique of *nāga kumbhaka*.

11. ***kūrma kumbhaka*** (KP-79)

When the blinking of the eyes is controlled and one becomes perfectly steady devoid of movement of the eyes and the whole body it is called *kūrma kumbhaka*. It brings steadiness of *vāyu* and the mind.

12. ***kṛkara kumbhaka*** (KP-80)

When there is a possibility of sneeze one should rub index and ring fingers with thumb. This controls sneeze and is known as *kṛkara kumbhaka*.

13. ***sahita kumbhaka*** (KP-85)

When *kumbhaka* is accompanied by *pūraka* and *recaka* it is termed as *sahita kumbhaka* which leads to *nāḍī-śuddhi* or purification of the *nāḍīs*.

14. ***agni-ṣoma kumbhaka*** (KP-87)

One should inhale through the right nostril, hold the breath as prescribed and exhale through the left nostril. Again inhale through the left nostril and after retaining the breath judiciously exhale through the right nostril. This is *agni-ṣoma kumbhaka.*

agni refers to right nostril and *soma* refers to left nostril.

15. ***sama kumbhaka*** (KP-99)

Without exhalation or inhalation one should mentally attend to the vital points like navel etc. This is called *sama kumbhaka.*

16. ***śānta-kumbhaka*** (KP-90)

When the breath is held internally or externally between the two vital points imagining its presence inside and outside, it is called *śānta-kumbhaka.*

It leads to *pratyāhāra* of nine vital points.

17. ***karṣaka kumbhaka*** (KP-100-103)

It is two-fold: *utkarṣaka* and *apakarṣaka.* In *utkarṣaka kumbhaka* one should hold the nose at its root and practise *pūraka, kumbhaka* and *recaka* according to the capacity.

In *apakarṣaka kumbhaka* one should partially close the nose during *pūraka* and *recaka.*

18. ***utkarṣaka-kumbhaka*** (KP-101)

See ***karṣaka-kumbhaka.***

19. ***apakarṣaka-kumbhaka*** (KP-102)

See ***karṣaka-kumbhaka.***

20. ***sahaja kumbhaka*** (KP-104)

Inhale the *prāṇa* through the nose carrying it along the *kuṇḍalī* and hold comfortably. Repeated practice of this is called *sahaja kumbhaka.*

21. ***dakṣiṇāvarta-cakra kumbhaka*** (KP-107)

Take the breath through *sūrya-nāḍī* (right nostril) and after retaining it in the chest, exhale through the *candra-nāḍi* (left nostril). Repeat this once again. This is *dakṣiṇāvarta-cakra kumbhaka.*

It is also called *sūrya-kumbhaka.*

22. ***vāmāvarta-cakra kumbhaka*** (KP-108)

It is just the reverse of the *dakṣiṇāvarta-cakra kumbhaka.*

23. ***dakṣiṇāvarta-śaṅkha-ku.*** (KP-106)

Take breath through right nostril, retain it and exhale through left nostril. Repeat this several times.

24. ***vāmāvarta-śaṅkha-ku.*** (KP-106)

Take breath through left nostril, retain it and exhale through right nostril. Repeat this several times.

25. ***gadā kumbhaka*** (KP-112, HTK)

Inhale through both the nostrils and after holding the breath exhale through the right nostril. This gives strength to the practitioner.

26. ***nāḍi-śuddhi kumbhaka*** (KP-114-117)

i) Inhale through one nostril and after holding the breath to capacity exhale through other nostril while contemplating on *haṃsa.* Again inhale through the nostril through which exhalation is done and after retaining the breath to the capacity, exhale through the opposite nostril. Repeat this process (KP-114).

ii) After inhaling through the right nostril, hold the breath while contemplating in the navel region on the orb of the mid-day sun of the summer. This leads to purification of the *nāḍīs* (KP-116).

iii) Inhale through the left nostril and while holding the breath visualize oozing of the nectar from the moon of the autumn night, situated in the lotus of thousand petals. This brings purification of the *nāḍīs* (KP-117).

27. ***śuddhi-kumbhaka (sūrya)*** (KP-116)
Inhale through right nostril and hold with concentration in the navel on the orb of the midday summer sun.

28. ***śuddhi-kumbhaka (candra)*** (KP-117)
Inhale through the left nostril and hold the breath while visualising on the oozing of the nectar from the moon of the autumn situated in the lotus of the thousand petals.

29. ***tatva kumbhaka*** (KP-122-125)
When a particular *tatva* is on the rise, one should practise *pūraka, kumbhaka* and *recaka.* Repeated practice leads to the control over that particular *tatva.* Thus, one attains control on all the five *tatvas.*

30. ***sūrya-bhedana kumbhaka*** (KP-127)
Inhale the outside air fully through the right nostril with sound and after holding it firmly, exhale through the *iḍā* or left nostril. This is *sūrya-bhedana* which removes diseases of abdomen caused by vitiated *vāta,* diseases of worms, chest, throat and brings purification of sinuses. It produces heat in the body.

31. ***candra-bhedana kumbhaka*** (KP-128)
This technique is just the opposite of *sūrya-bhedana.* One inhales through the left nostril and exhales through the right nostril after holding the breath.

This *candra-bhedana kumbhaka* produces cold in the body and is nourishing.

32. ***ujjāyī kumbhaka*** (KP-132)

With closed mouth inhale through the two nostrils. Then hold the breath judiciously and exhale through the left nostril. This can be practised any time.

In this text, there is no mention of frictional sound produced during inhalation or exhalation as is mentioned in HP-II.51.

33. ***kumbharāja*** (KP-134)

One should forcefully inhale the air and hold the breath by closing the nose to the capacity before one exhales.

It brings control over the *vāyu* and increases the heat.

34. ***śītalī ku.*** (KP-136)

A synonym for *sīt-kārī kumbhaka.*

35. ***sīt-kārī kumbhaka*** (KP-136-140)

Raise the tongue and inhale the air making '*sīt*' sound. Hold the breath and exhale through the nose.

It helps to control hunger, thirst, sleep, laziness and one becomes free from all problems of health.

36. ***kāka-cañcu kumbhaka*** (KP-137-148)

i) Turning the tongue upward, take the air in through the mouth producing '*sīt*' sound. Hold the breath and then exhale through both the nostrils while concentrating on the sound produced. This is called *sīt-kārī kumbhaka* (KP-137-138).

ii) Forming the tongue into a tube take the air in through it. After holding the breath exhale through the nose. This is known as *kāka-cañcuka* (KP-141).

iii) Forming the mouth like the beak of a crow, take the air in and hold it. By raising the tongue taste the flow of nectar and then exhale through both the nostrils. This is called *sīt-kārī-kāka-cañcuka* (KP-143).

iv) By pressing the teeth together, take the air slowly through the mouth and after holding the breath with upturned tongue exhale through the nose. This is *kāka-cañcuka* according to *kākudaśravā* (KP-148).

37. ***śītalī-kāka-cañcu kumbhaka*** (KP-143)
See *kāka-cañcu-kumbhaka* above.

38. ***mātrā kumbhaka*** (KP-153)
When particular time units are used during *kumbhaka* it becomes *mātrā kumbhaka*.

Different varieties are described in the text which are noted below :-

i. Inhale for 16 *mātrās*, retain the breath for 64 *mātrās* and exhale for 32 *mātrās*.

When it is practised with concentration on navel region it generates heat, on *svādhiṣṭhāna*, it increases flow of nectar, on *mūlādhāra*, it removes indigestion.

ii. Hold the breath without force for a period of two *palas* (48 seconds) or for the time taken for recitation of five long vowels, after inhaling for half the period of *kumbhaka* and exhale for the same period of inhalation.

iii. *mātrā-kumbhaka* is progressively practised with 12 *mātrās* or 25 *palas* for *kumbhaka* in the first variety, *kumbhaka* for 50 *palas* in the second variety and 75 *palas* in the third variety.

The last one is according to the tradition of *dattātreya*.

39. ***bhūta-śuddhi kumbhaka*** (KP-157)
When *mātrā kumbhaka* is practised with progressive concentration on all the six regions (of *cakras*), it leads to purification and balance of the five *bhūtas*.

40. ***bhastrikā kumbhaka*** (KP-164-168)

Three types of *bhastrikā kumbhaka* have been described in the text.

i) Rapidly exhale and inhale like the bellows of the blacksmith until fatigue sets in. Then inhale through the right nostril, hold the breath with *jālandhara bandha* and exhale through the left nostril.

ii) Hold the tip of the nose with hand and closing the left nostril inhale through the right nostril and quickly exhale through the left by closing the right nostril. Repeat this several times. Then inhale through the right nostril, retain the breath with *jālandhara bandha* and exhale through the left nostril. This is called *antar-bhastrā* (KP-167).

iii) Exhale and inhale quickly through both the nostrils. Then after holding the breath exhale through the nose. This is called *antaraṅga-bhastrikā.*

iv) In his commentary on HP-II.64, *brahmānanda* describes a variety of *bhastrikā* as follows :

Close the left nostril and rapidly and forcefully exhale and inhale several times. Then inhale through right nostril, hold the breath to the capacity and exhale through the left nostril. After this, close the right nostril and rapidly exhale and inhale several times through left nostril. Then inhale through left nostril, hold the breath to the capacity and exhale through the right nostril.

41. ***antaraṅga-ku.*** (KP-168)

Retain the breath after sudden exhalation and inhalation.

42. ***bhrāmarī-kumbhaka*** (KP-169)

Inhale rapidly producing the sound of a black bee and after retaining the breath exhale slowly with the sound of a black bee. This is *bhrāmarī-kumbhaka* which produces ecstasy.

43. ***mūrcchanā kumbhaka*** (KP-170)

Hold the breath after complete inhalation and while adopting *jālandhara-bandha*, exhale. This is *mūrcchanā kumbhaka* which brings pleasant mental stupor.

44. ***plāvinī kumbhaka*** (KP-171)

After taking the breath fully and adopting *jālandhara-bandha* lie on the water which causes floating on the water. This is *plāvinī kumbhaka.*

45. ***svaṅga śṛṅkhalā*** (KP-176-178)

One should inhale the air followed by the retention and again and again try to inhale and retain repeatedly until one is exhausted.

One should then practise *pūraka* followed by the *pūraka* again.

Similarly one should retain the breath to the maximum capacity before exhalation.

One should exhale and hold the breath, followed by exhalation and retention again and again as per the instruction of the *guru*. This should not be practised without the *haṃsa-vedha*.

46. ***kumbhāntara śṛṅkhalā*** (KP-183)

kumbhaka followed by the *kumbhaka* as instructed by the *guru* is the technique called *kumbhāntara śṛṅkhalā*.

47. ***jīvacāla*** (KP-184-185)

During *kumbhaka* one should activate *prāṇa vāyu* in upward and downward directions.

48. ***ṣaḍaṅga kumbhaka*** (KP-187)

mūlabandha, pūraka, jālandhara-bandha, kumbhaka, uḍḍiyāna and *recaka* are the six components of *ṣaḍaṅga kumbhaka* proclaimed by *śambhu*.

49. ***kamala kumbhaka*** (KP-189)

Inhale through the *śurya nāḍī* and after holding the breath exhale through the *candra nāḍī*. This is called *kamala kumbhaka*. It is the same as *sūrya-bhedana kumbhaka*.

50. ***kumuda kumbhaka*** (KP-190)

Inhale through the left nostril and after retaining the breath exhale through both the nostrils.

51. ***krama-netra-ku.*** (KP-191)

Inhale quickly through right nostril. Hold the breath and then inhale through left nostril. After holding the breath exhale in the same order (***krama***) . This can also be reversed (***vyutkrama***).

52. ***netra-kumbhaka*** (KP-191)

Inhale through the right nostril, hold the breath. Again inhale through the left, hold the breath with effort and exhale in the similar sequence. This is known as *netra kumbhaka* and may be practised both in inverse (***krama)*** and reverse (***vyutkrama***) orders.

53. ***trinetra-kumbhaka*** (KP-192)

Inhale quickly through the left nostril and hold the breath followed by inhalation through the right nostril and retain the breath. Then inhale the breath again through both the nostrils, hold the breath systematically before exhalation. This is called *tri-netra-kumbhaka* after *śiva* (*tri-netra*-- a synonym of *śiva)*.

54. ***triśūla-kumbhaka*** (KP-193)

Inhale through the nose and mouth simultaneously and hold the breath before exhalation.

55. ***eka-meru kumbhaka*** (KP-206)

When the period of *kumbhaka* increases with the knowledge of internal and external movements of *prāṇa* or determining the number of *mātrās*, respirations or with devotion to God, it is called *eka-meru.*

56. ***dvi-meru kumbhaka*** (KP-207)

With the increase of *pūraka* it becomes *dvi-meru kumbhaka.*

57. ***tri-meru-kumbhaka*** (KP-207)

With the increase of *recaka* it becomes *tri-meru kumbhaka.*

58. ***ghaṭi-bandha-ku.*** (KP-211)

One should tie up the joint of an hourglass made of copper with a hole at the bottom and fill it with sand and use it for measurement of time.

Apart from the *kumbhakas* mentioned in the KP, some *kumbhakas* are found described in other texts. They are described here for the benefit of the readers.

59. ***kālāgni kumbhaka*** (HSC)

prāṇa has a tendency to move out. When this tendency is reversed, that is, when it is not allowed to go out by holding it inside, it is called *kālāgni kumbhaka.*

60. ***nāda kumbhaka*** or ***lambā guru prāṇāyāma*** (HSC)

Sit straight in *padmāsana.* Inhale deeply and produce the sound of *om* in a low tone and lengthened to the extent so that one feels it rising from the navel and getting the vibrations from heart and throat and reaching upto the *brahma-randhra.* Repeat this several times for the prolongation of *kumbhaka.*

61. ***utkrānti-prāṇāyāma*** (HTK-ch.53)

At the time of willfully leaving the body, a *yogī* assumes *vīrāsana* and inhales through the left nostril. He pulls *prāṇa* along with *ātmā* upwards through *suṣumnā.*

62. ***vāma-gati*** or ***vartma-gati kumbhaka*** (HSC, HTK-X.28)

Inhale through both the nostrils and after holding the breath appropriately, exhale through both the nostrils. This is called *vāma-gati kumbhaka.*

The same is described as *vartma-gati kumbhaka* by HTK-X.28.

63. ***bhujaṅgī-karaṇa kumbhaka*** (HR-II.32)

Swallow the air by the throat and after holding the breath, expel the air through the throat. This is *bhujaṅgī-karaṇa.*

64. ***bhuyaṅgama-kumbhaka*** (JP-V.487-490)

Sit in *vīrāsana.* Raise the tongue slightly and bring it little outside. Then inhale, hold the breath to the capacity and exhale through the tongue. Apply all the *bandhas.* Direct the gaze to the tip of the nose. This is *bhuyaṅgama kumbhaka.*

65. ***trāṭaka kumbhaka*** (JP-V.491-493)

Sit in *bhadrāsana.* Turn the tongue upwards. Inhale through the nose, retain the breath and exhale through the nose. Adopt all the *bandhas.* This is *trāṭaka-kumbhaka* which brings purification of *nāḍīs.*

66. ***kaṇṭhi-vetālī kumbhaka*** (JP-V.494-498)

Assume *ardha-siddhāsana* by placing the left heel under the anus and right foot on the left thigh. Then inhale and hold the breath in the throat and exhale through the nose.

This *kaṇṭhi-vetālī-kumbhaka* should be practised in the summer. After six months of practice all the *nāḍīs* get purified.

67. ***bhoralikā*** (JP-V.477-481)

Adopt *baddha-padmāsana.* Take the air in through the navel to the limit while producing sound of a black bee. Do not close the nose. Repeat this several times. This resembles *bhrāmarī.*

68. ***kevalī-kumbhaka*** (GŚ)

Draw the air in through both the nostrils and hold the breath. Mentally recite *soham mantra* at the rate of 15 per minute before exhalation.

69. ***śūnyaka-kumbhaka*** (SauP-XII. 22-24)

After exhalation hold the breath outside without inhaling the air. Contemplate on the moon inside and absorb the nectar oozing from it.

70. ***kevala-kumbhaka*** (retention of breath irrespective of inhalation or exhalaṭion)

When the breath is automatically held without prior inhalation or exhalation it is called *kevala-kumbhaka.* Other synonyms for this are *stambha-vṛtti, saṅghaṭṭa-karaṇa, śānta* and *sama.*

kumbhakas are broadly divided into *sahita* and *kevala. ābhyantara* and *bāhya-kumbhakas* come under the category of *ṣahita.* All the *kumbhakas* are called *ameru* as against *meru* which is *kevala.*

sahita-kumbhakas are divided into *agarbha* and *sagarbha. agarbha* is also called *nigarbha* by GŚ in which there is no use of *mantra* or meditation.

sagarbha varieties are, on the other hand, always accompanied by repetition of *mantras* and some kind of meditation.

sagarbha-kumbhaka again is classified as *sadhūma, vidhūma, sajvāla, praśānta, salakṣya* and *alakṣya* which involve different kinds of visualizations or meditations.

Some other techniques of *prāṇāyāma* available in YRah(N) are noted below:

1. ***āndolī-prāṇāyāma*** (YRah(N)-I.100)
One rolls the tongue while breathing.

2. ***laharī-prāṇāyāma*** (YRah(N)-I.100)
Breath with short inhalation and exhalation, first through one nostril and then through the other.

3. ***kapālabhāti-prāṇāyāma*** (YRah(N)-I.100)
Take short and fast breaths while moving the abdomen in and out.

Although there are different *kumbhakas* and they have been described with different names in the text of KP, many varieties of *kumbhaka* have similar techniques. As the author says, "*saṃjñā-bhedo na vāstavaḥ*" (they differ only in names, not in factual technique).

In spite of description of various *kumbhakas*, the author is loud in praise of *ameru* and *meru kumbhakas*. He talks of *eka-meru, dvi-meru* and *tri-meru kumbhakas*. But what is most important is the various stages in the attainment of the *meru kumbhaka*.

These stages have been described as 47 and they include all the levels of spiritual development.

These 47 stages (*bhūmis*) are mentioned as follows :-

sparśā, mūḍhā, sthāna-vāhā, dhātu-śoṣaṇā, puṣṭidā, jitāsanā, anāhatā, śubhāśubhā, smaraharā, mārgadā, śakti-bodhinī, śakti-cālanā, citta-kampā, jitāsanā, jyotiṣmatī, mātrā-prakāśā, gandhavati, rasapradā, rūpa-grāhaṇa-kāriṇi, sparśavatikā, śabda-suśruti, buddhidā, śruti-bodhanā, jayā, vāk-siddhidā, citra-darśanā, vegavati, manojava-dāyinī, gati-pradā, aṇimā, laghimā, prāpti, prākāmya, mahimā, īśitvam, vaśitvam, kāmāvasāyitā, nivartikā, bhūmayī, toyamayī, tejomayī, vāyumayī, vyomamayī, pradhāna-jaya-dāyinī, viveka-khyāti, dharma-megha, brahma-mayī or *paramātma-prakāśabhū.*

These stages are a continuum of experiences that the *yogī* passes through as a result of the continuous practice of *kumbhaka.*

These stages are not found mentioned in any available text. Therefore, it is the unique feature of KP.

Some observations about the text

i. Traditionally *āsanas* are practised before one takes up the technique of *kumbhaka.* PYS-II.49 indicates this.

Chronic muscular tensions prevent full natural respiration and so decrease the energy level. Through *āsanas,* one could remove muscular tensions thus facilitating respiration.

However, the importance of the contribution of *āsanas* has not been emphasized in the KP.

ii. Although, holding of breath is a significant phase of *prāṇāyāma,* the supplementary and complementary phases of *pūraka* and *recaka* are differently practised in different *prāṇāyāmas* as can be seen from the following table presented overleaf:

INSPIRATORY-EXPIRATORY PATTERN IN DIFFERENT VARIETIES OF KUMBHAKA

Name of the variety of *prāṇayāma*	Inspiration through	Expiration through
1. *sūrya-bhedana*	Right nostril	Left nostril
2. *ujjāyī*	Both nostrils	Left nostril
3. *śitalī*	Tongue	Both nostrils
4. *sītkārī*	Mouth	Both nostrils
5. *bhastrikā*	Right nostril (after *kapāla-bhāti* type of forceful and fast inspiration and expiration through both the nostrils)	Both nostrils
6. *bhrāmarī*	Both nostrils (while producing the humming sound of bee)	Both nostrils
7. *mūrcchā*	Both nostrils	Both nostrils (while maintaining *jālandhara bandha*)
8. *plāvinī*	Both nostrils (after filling the stomach with air)	Both nostrils

iii. Different types of *pūraka* and *recaka* have been described in the text of KP. But there is no mention about what type of *pūraka* and *recaka* should be used with *kumbhakas*.

iv. Preliminary preparations through *kriyās* is not mentioned. Although *nāḍī-śuddhi* is discussed, it is through the various techniques of *prāṇayāma*.

v. It is emphasized that the *kumbhaka* should be accompanied by concentration.

vi. In this text, *kumbhaka* does not necessarily mean holding of breath, but it also includes the technique of concentration and visualization.

vii. There is no mention of closing the nose in all the *kumbhakas*.

viii. Application of *bandhas* is mentioned only in selected *kumbhakas*.

ix. Many-a-time it is seen that all the three phases of *pūraka*, *kumbhaka* and *recaka* are not mentioned in the description of the technique.

x. The author refers to *śārīra* in which he has already discussed *agarbha* and *sagarbha*. It is not clear whether this '*śārīra*' is his earlier work or else. He has discussed *agarbha* and *sagarbha* earlier in some work, but not in the present text.

Dr. M. L. Gharote
Dr. Parimal Devnath

कुम्भकपद्धतिः
kumbhaka-paddhatiḥ

श्रीगणेशाय नमः ॥

śrīgaṇeśāya namaḥ ॥

Tr. Salutation to *śrīgaṇeśa.*

श्रीगुरुं सच्चिदानन्दं सर्वात्मानमजं विभुम् ।
क्लेशकर्मविपाकादिरहितं समुपास्महे[1] ॥ १ ॥

śrī-guruṃ saccidānandaṃ sarvātmānam-ajaṃ vibhum ।
kleśa-karma-vipākādi-rahitaṃ samupāsmahe ॥ 1 ॥

Tr. I bow down to *śrī-guru* who is Eternal-Conscious-Bliss, essence of all, unborn, omnipresent, devoid of afflictions, unaffected by *karma* (actions) and their results. 1.

स्वयत्न्या चेष्टया युक्तो व्याप्य देहं स्थितोऽनिलः[2] ।
जगत्सूत्रात्मने तस्मै नमः कालामृतात्मने ॥ २ ॥

sva-yatnyā ceṣṭayā yukto vyāpya dehaṃ sthito'nilaḥ ।
jagat-sūtrātmane tasmai namaḥ kālāmṛtātmane ॥ 2 ॥

Tr. The vital air (*prāṇa*), by its own effort, pervades the whole body. I bow down to that source of the creation, which is the essence, time (*kāla*) and immortal. 2.

कुत्सगोत्रसमुद्भूतमुदीच्यं काशिकाश्रयम् ।
[3]शिवरामाह्वयं तातं राजकुलमुपास्महे ॥ ३ ॥

kutsa-gotra-samudbhūtam-udīcyaṃ kāśikāśrayam ।
śivarāmāhvayaṃ tātaṃ rājakulam-upāsmahe ॥ 3 ॥

Tr. I bow down to my father named *śivarāma* of *kutsa* clan, belonging to *udīcya brāhmaṇa*, who hails from a royal family residing in *kāśī* (Benaras). 3.

Note. After salutation to the deity and *guru* the author gives information about himself. From this information we could only know that he was a resident of *kāśī* (Benaras) and came from the royal family of *śivarāma*, his father, of *kutsa*-clan (*gotra*)

---

1. समुस्महे –J. 2. ऽनलः–J. 3. राजकुल्डाो रघुपतिः कुर्वे कुम्भकपद्धतिम् – extra in A.

of *udīcya brāhmaṇa.* From the variat reading of A, we gather that the author's another name is *raghupati.* He also seems to be the author of *sat-karma-saṅgraha.* 1-3.

योगग्रन्थसहस्राणां सारमाकृष्य यत्नतः ।
सम्प्रदायानुसारेण कुर्मः कुम्भकपद्धतिम् ॥ ४ ॥
yoga-grantha-sahasrāṇām sāram-ākṛṣya yatnataḥ ।
sampradāyānusāreṇa kūrmaḥ kumbhaka-paddhatim ॥ 4 ॥

Tr. I am compiling this *kumbhaka-paddhati* which is based on the essence of several *yogic* treatises and following the tradition. 4.

Note. The author calls his treatise "*kumbhaka-paddhati*". As is pointed out, this "*kumbhaka-paddhati*" is based on tradition and information contained in several *yoga* treatises. 4.

निरावरणकं ज्योतिः सार्वज्ञं दीर्घजीविनम् ।
सिद्धिः सर्वविधाभ्यासात् प्राणायामस्य जायते ॥ ५ ॥
nirāvaraṇakaṃ jyotiḥ sārvajñaṃ dīrgha-jīvinam ।
siddhiḥ sarva-vidhābhyāsāt prāṇāyāmasya jāyate ॥ 5 ॥

Tr. With the accomplishment of all round practices of *prāṇāyāma*, one perceives effulgent light, becomes omniscient and attains longevity. 5.

Note. Here the author uses the word *prāṇāyāma* as a synonym for *kumbhaka*. 5.

श्रीगुरोः कृपया लब्धः हंसवेधो जितेन्द्रियः ।
पूजिताखिलनाथो य ईशयोगेन दीक्षितः ॥ ६ ॥[1]
śrī-guroḥ kṛpayā labdhaḥ haṃsavedho jitendriyaḥ ।
pūjitākhila-nātho ya īśa-yogena dīkṣitaḥ ॥ 6 ॥

Tr. I received *haṃsa-vedha* by the grace of *guru* who is self-restrained, respected by all the *nāthas* and who was initiated by the grace of *īśa* (God). 6.

Note. The *haṃsa-vedha* referred to here has not been explained in the text. (See note on verse KP-179). 6.

प्रविष्टो मण्डलं योगी लब्धपूरककुम्भकः ।
प्राणायामं ततः कुर्यादन्यथा क्लेशभाग् भवेत् ॥ ७ ॥[1]

1. Verse not in A.

praviṣṭo maṇḍalaṃ yogī labdha-pūraka-kumbhakaḥ ।
prāṇāyāmaṃ tataḥ kuryād-anyathā kleśa-bhāg-bhavet ।7।

Tr. A *yogī* having been initiated in a tradition and only after receiving the technique of *pūraka* and *kumbhaka* should practise *prāṇāyāma.* Otherwise he may face troubles.7.

अथातः सम्प्रवक्ष्यामि कुम्भमार्गं शिवोदितम् ॥ ८ ॥[1]
athātaḥ sampravakṣyāmi kumbhamārgaṃ śivoditam ॥ 8 ॥

Tr. Now I shall narrate the technique of *kumbhaka* as handed down by *śiva.* 8.

Note. The author emphasizes on the origin of *kumbhaka* tradition from *śiva* himself. Here "*kumbha-mārga*" seems to be a synonym for "*kumbhaka-paddhati*" . 8.

वक्त्रं नासायुगं मार्गाः प्राणपूरकरेचयोः ।
नासापुटयुगे चापि पञ्चतत्वविभेदतः ॥
नाडीवक्त्रादिरन्ध्राणां ज्ञेयाः सूक्ष्माः शिवोदिताः ॥ ९ ॥
vaktraṃ nāsāyugaṃ mārgāḥ prāṇa-pūraka-recayoḥ ।
nāsāpuṭa-yuge cāpi pañca-tatva-vibhedataḥ ॥
nāḍī-vaktrādi-randhrāṇāṃ jñeyāḥ sūkṣmāḥ śivoditāḥ ॥9॥

Tr. Mouth and nostrils are the only passages of *prāṇa* for entry and exit. When the *prāṇa* enters through nasal passage, it gets manifested into five elements, and moves through the openings of the different *nāḍīs*, subtlety of which should be known from the narration of *śiva.* 9.

स्वतो निःसरणं कोष्ठ्यवायोः प्रश्वास उच्यते ।
तथा प्रवेशः[2] श्वासः स्यादिति पातञ्जलाः[3] जगुः ॥ १० ॥
svato niḥsaraṇaṃ koṣṭhya-vāyoḥ praśvāsa ucyate ।
tathā praveśaḥ śvāsaḥ syād-iti pātañjalāḥ jaguḥ ॥ 10 ॥

Tr. According to the school of *patañjali*, passing out of the air from the chest cavity is called *praśvāsa* (exhalation) and entering in of the air is called *śvāsa* (inhalation). 10.

---

1. Verse not in A. 2. प्रवेश–J. 3. पातञ्जला–J.

Noteุ. Commenting on the *sūtra* –"*tasmin sati śvāsa-praśvāsayor-gati-vicchedaḥ prāṇāyāmaḥ*" (PYS-II.49), *vyāsa* explains the term `*śvāsa*' as taking the external air in (inhalation) and `*praśvāsa*' as expelling the air out from the chest (exhalation) (see also in VB-I.31). 10.

उन्मुखस्तु भवेत् प्राणोऽधोमुखोऽपानतां व्रजेत् ।
एष एव इति प्राह भुशुण्ड[1]श्चिरजीवनः ॥ ११ ॥
unmukhas-tu bhavet prāṇo'dhomukho'pānatām vrajet ।
eṣa eva iti prāha bhuśuṇḍaś-cira-jīvanaḥ ॥ 11 ॥

Tr. *prāṇa* has upward movement while *apāna* has downward movement. This has been narrated by *bhuśuṇḍa* who lived long. 11.

श्वासप्रश्वासकृद्वायुरधऊर्ध्वं प्रधावति ।
देहेऽखण्डोऽप्यपानः[2] स्यादधोगमनकर्मकृत् ॥
देहोर्ध्वभागसञ्चारकरणात् प्राण उच्यते ॥ १२ ॥
śvāsa-praśvāsa-kṛd-vāyur-adha-ūrdhvaṃ pradhāvati ।
dehe'khaṇḍo'pyapānaḥ syād-adhogamana-karmakṛt ॥
dehordhvabhāga-sañcāra-karaṇāt prāṇa ucyate ॥ 12 ॥

Tr. The *vāyu* which causes *śvāsa* (inhalation) and *praśvāsa* (exhalation), moves downwards and upwards respectively. In the body, *apāna* acts all the time moving downwards, while because of the upward movement, it is called *prāṇa*. 12.

Note. The word *prāṇa* etymologically means `*pra*'+`*an*', which means `moving upwards'. 12.

पूर्वोत्तरार्द्धभेदेन चन्द्रसूर्याविमावपि ।
इडापिंगलयोश्चारादित्यप्याहुर्महर्षयः ॥ १३ ॥
pūrvottarārdha-bhedena candra-sūryāvimāvapi ।
iḍā-piṅgalayoś-cārād-ityapyāhur-maharṣayaḥ ॥ 13 ॥

Tr. The place of *candra* and *sūrya* is located in the upper and lower regions respectively. According to the *maharṣis* (sages), place of *candra* and *sūrya* is associated with the working of *iḍā* and *piṅgalā* respectively. 13.

---

1. भुशुन्द्र–J. 2. प्यपान–J.

वामामिडां चरन् वायुः[1] रात्रीन्द्वमृतसंज्ञितः ।
क्ष्वेडार्क्कार्ह्वां समानाह्वः स्याद् दक्षां पिंगलां चरन् ॥१४॥

vāmām-iḍāṃ caran vāyuḥ
rātrīndvamṛta-sañjitaḥ ॥
kṣveḍārkkāhvāṃ samānāhvaḥ
syād dakṣāṃ piṅgalāṃ caran ॥ 14 ॥

Tr. The movement of the *vāyu (prāṇa)* in the left *iḍā nāḍī* is called *rātri* (night), *indu* (moon) and *amṛta* (nectar). The movement of the *vāyu* in the right *nāḍī piṅgalā* is called *kṣveḍā* (poison), *arka* (sun) and *ahan* (day). 14.

श्वासप्रश्वासयोर्यत्र गतिविच्छेदनं भवेत् ।
सामान्यलक्षणं प्रोक्तं प्राणायामस्य चासने ॥ १५ ॥

śvāsa-praśvāsayor-yatra gati-vicchedanaṃ bhavet ।
sāmānya-lakṣaṇaṃ proktaṃ prāṇāyāmasya cāsane ॥ 15 ॥

Tr. A pause in the movement of inhalation and exhalation is the general characteristic of *prāṇayāma* during *āsana.* 15.

Note. This *prāṇāyāma* refers to *upaniṣadic* variety, in which the three stages of *prānāyāma* namely- *pūraka, kumbhaka* and *recaka* are integrated with `*a*', `*u*' and `*m*'- the three letters of `*OM*' *(praṇava*). 15.

प्राणायामस्त्रिभिः प्रोक्तो रेचकपूरकुम्भकैः ॥ १६ ॥

prāṇāyāmas-tribhiḥ prokto recaka-pūra-kumbhakaiḥ ।16।

Tr. *prāṇāyāma* is described as three-fold, namely, *recaka, pūraka* and *kumbhaka.* 16.

Note. According to SSP-II.35, it is of four types including *saṅghaṭṭa-karaṇa* which is a synonym for *kevala-kumbhaka.* 16.

अकारः पूरकः कुम्भ उकारो रेचकस्तु मः ।
प्रणवात्मकता चैवं प्राणायामस्य कीर्त्तिता ॥ १७ ॥

akāraḥ pūrakaḥ kumbha ukāro recakas-tu maḥ ।
praṇavātmakatā caivaṃ prāṇāyāmasya kīrtitā ॥ 17 ॥

Tr. The nature of *prāṇāyāma* has been described as *praṇava*, where *pūraka* represents `*a*', *kumbhaka* `*u*' and *recaka* `*ma*'. 17.

---

1. वायु -J.

निसर्गसिद्धे मात्रात्वं मुनिभिस्तत्र तत्वतः ॥ १८ ॥
nisargasiddhe mātrātvaṃ munibhis-tatra tatvataḥ ॥ 18 ॥

Tr. Sages have determined *mātrā* basically on natural flow of breath. 18.

Note. `*nisarga-siddha mātrā*' refers to the natural breathing. 18.

बाह्यगं घोणमाप्राणं पूरयेदाननेन वा ।
निरोधः पूरकः प्रोक्तः कृष्णद्वैपायनादिभिः ॥
तथान्तर्गामिनं प्राणं रेचयेत् स तु रेचकः ॥ १९ ॥
bāhyagaṃ ghoṇam-āprāṇaṃ pūryed-ānanena vā ।
nirodhaḥ pūrakaḥ proktaḥ kṛṣṇadvaipāyanādibhiḥ ॥
tathāntargāminaṃ prāṇaṃ recayet sa tu recakaḥ ॥ 19 ॥

Tr. When external *prāṇa* is inhaled through either nose or mouth is called *nirodha-pūraka* by the authorities like *kṛṣṇa-dvaipāyana*. Similarly, when the inhaled *prāṇa* is exhaled, it is called *recaka*. 19.

Note. *kṛṣṇa-dvaipāyana—* another name of *vyāsa*, was the son of *satyavatī* and *parāśara*. His well-known compositions are *brahma-sūtras* and *purāṇas*.

Commenting on PYS-I.34, *vyāsa* defines *recaka* as follows- `*kauṣṭhyasya vāyor-nāsikā-puṭābhyāṃ prayatna-viśeṣād-vamanaṃ pracchardanam*'- i.e. effortful expulsion of air from the (chest) cavity is called *recaka*.

According to *yogacandrikā* quoted by HTK-38:77-78, when *prāṇa* moves inside coming from outside up to 12 digits and touches inside (the nose), it is called *pūraka*. From 12 digits outside (*prāṇa*) gets in the body by causing a touch in organs which is considered *pūraka*. 19.

प्राणं यत्राचलं कृत्वा धारयेद्यत्नवान् मुनिः ।
स एष कुम्भको नाम सर्वयोगिनिषेवितः ॥ २० ॥
prāṇaṃ yatrācalaṃ kṛtvā dhārayed-yatnavān muniḥ ।
sa eṣa kumbhako nāma sarva-yogi-niṣevitaḥ ॥ 20 ॥

Tr. When a *muni* effortfully holds the *prāṇa* without movement, it is called *kumbhaka*, which is practised by all the *yogīs*. 20.

पूरमाभ्यन्तरं शेषो रेकं बाह्यं प्रचक्ष्यते ।
कुम्भकः स्तम्भ इत्याख्यः संज्ञाभेदो न वास्तवः ॥ २१ ॥
pūram-ābhyantaraṃ śeṣo rekaṃ bāhyaṃ pracakṣyate ।
kumbhakaḥ stambha ityākhyaḥ sañjābhedo na vāstavaḥ।21।

Tr. *pūraka*, *recaka* and *kumbhaka* are synonyms of *ābhyantara*, *bāhya* and *stambha*. The difference lies only in terms and not in practice. 21.

Note. *pūraka*, *kumbhaka* and *recaka* are the general terms used in connection with *prāṇāyāma*, especially in the *haṭha-yogic* tradition. However, here *pūraka* and *recaka* have been used synonymously for *prāṇāyāma*, the characteristic of which is holding of breath. The terms *ābhyantara* (internal), *bāhya* (external) and *stambha* (retention) come from PYS-II.50. They have been used in the text synonymously for the variety of *prāṇāyāma (kumbhaka)*. 19-21.

इति सामान्यलक्षणोक्तं[1] विशेषः कश्चिदीर्यते ॥ २२ ॥
iti sāmānya-lakṣaṇoktaṃ viśeṣaḥ kaś-cid-īryate ॥ 22 ॥

Tr. These are general characteristics. Some special characteristics are being explained further. 22.

द्वादशांगुलबाह्यस्य श्वासः स्वाभिमुखो यदा ।
स बाह्यपूरकः प्रोक्तो भालनेत्रेण योगिना ॥
हृदि क्रमतः आपूर्य बाह्याभ्यन्तरपूरकः ॥ २३ ॥
dvādaśāṅgula-bāhyasya śvāsaḥ svābhimukho yadā ।
sa bāhya-pūrakaḥ prokto bhālanetreṇa yoginā ॥
hṛdi kramataḥ āpūrya bāhyābhyantara-pūrakaḥ ॥ 23 ॥

Tr. The breath moving into the nose from a distance of twelve *aṅgulas* (digits—nine inches) is called *bāhya-pūraka* by *yogī bhāla-netra (śiva)*. That which moves in the chest is called *bāhyābhyantara-pūraka*. 23.

सौषुम्णारन्ध्रं प्रविशेत् पूरितश्चेत् समीरणः ।
स एष शिवसम्प्रोक्तः पूरकश्चान्तराख्यकः[2] ॥ २४ ॥
sauṣumṇā-randhraṃ praviśet pūritaś-cet samīraṇaḥ ।
sa eṣa śiva-samproktaḥ pūrakaś-cāntarākhyakaḥ ॥ 24 ॥

---

1. लक्ष्मीक्तं–J. 2. पूरकश्चान्तरान्तरः–A.

Tr. When inhaled air enters the opening of *suṣumṇā*, it is called *antara-pūraka* by *śiva*. 24.

सौषुम्णविवराद् वायोर्निर्गममन्तररेचकः[1] ॥ २५ ॥
sauṣumṇa-vivarād vāyor-nirgamam-antara-recakaḥ ॥25॥

Tr. When the *vāyu* goes out of the opening of *suṣumṇā*, it is *antara-recaka*. 25.

हृत्स्थानान्निर्गतो वायुर्नासान्तं प्रव्रजेद् यदा ।
भवेन गदितः सोऽयं बाह्याभ्यन्तररेचकः ॥ २६ ॥
hṛt-shtānān-nirgato vāyur-nāsāntaṃ pravrajed yadā ।
bhavena gaditaḥ so'yaṃ bāhyābhyantara-recakaḥ ॥ 26 ॥

Tr. When the *vāyu* moves up to the end of the nostrils from the thoracic cavity, it is called *bāhyābhyantara-recaka* by *bhava (śiva)*. 26.

नासाग्रादपि निर्गत्य द्वादशांगुलसम्मिते ।
व्योम्नि याते खगे प्राह शंकरो बाह्यरेचकम् ॥ २७ ॥
nāsāgrād-api nirgatya dvādaśāṅgula-sammite ।
vyomni yāte khage prāha śaṅkaro bāhya-recakam ॥ 27 ॥

Tr. When the *prāṇa* moves in the space up to twelve digits (nine inches) from the tip of the nose, it is called *bāhya-recaka* by *śaṅkara*. 27.

Note. The process of *pūraka* and *recaka* has been meticulously analyzed and described in this text which is not found in any other text. Also see HTK-38:73. 23-27.

सुषुम्णान्तर्गतं तस्यां निर्विकल्पेन चेतसा ।
धारयेन्मारुतं योगी सोऽन्तःकुम्भः शिवोदितः ॥ २८ ॥
suṣumṇāntargataṃ tasyāṃ nirvikalpena cetasā ।
dhārayen-mārutaṃ yogī so'ntaḥ-kumbhaḥ śivoditaḥ ।28।

Tr. When the *mārut (prāṇa)* is retained in *suṣumṇā* without any mental distraction by a *yogī*, it is called *antaḥ-kumbhaka* by *śiva*. 28.

1. निर्गमं तररेच्चकः–J.

शरीरे पूरितं वायुं कोष्ठे सम्यग्निरोधयेत् ।
सुषुम्णारहितं चापि बाह्याभ्यन्तरकुम्भकः ॥ २९ ॥

śarīre pūritaṃ vāyuṃ koṣṭhe samyag-nirodhayet ।
suṣumṇārahitaṃ cāpi bāhyābhyantara-kumbhakaḥ ॥ 29 ॥

Tr. When inhaled air is properly retained in the chest cavity without reference to *suṣumṇā*, it is called *bāhyābhyantara-kumbhaka*. 29.

पूरितोऽयं विनिर्द्दिष्टो देवलादिमुनीश्वरैः ॥ ३० ॥

pūrito'yaṃ vinirddiṣṭo devalādi-munīśvaraiḥ ॥ 30 ॥

Tr. The same is called *pūrita* by *munis* like *devala*. 30.

Note. *devala* is described as an important ancient *ṛṣi* and a *smṛti-kāra* (an exponent of the canonical texts). His quotations are profusely scattered in various texts on the *dharma-śāstra*. There are many quotations on the religious and *yogic* practices attributed to him. He elaborately describes *prāṇāyāma* from *smārta* point of view. Classical texts written on *yājñyavalkya* namely, *mitākṣarā, aparārka, smṛticandrikā* quote *devala*. *devala* was a contemporary of other *smṛtikāras* like *bṛhaspati, kātyāyana* etc.

dharmadīpa is a compilation of 300 *ślokas* composed by *devala* which throw light on the diversity and vastness of *smṛti* literature. 30.

रेचयित्वा बहिर्वायुं बाह्याकाशे क्रमेण यत् ।
धारयेत् प्रयतो योगी बहिःकुम्भस्तु रेचितः ॥ ३१ ॥

recayitvā bahir-vāyuṃ bāhyākāśe krameṇa yat ।
dhārayet prayato yogī bahiḥ-kumbhastu recitaḥ ॥ 31 ॥

Tr. When the air is exhaled slowly and breath is retained outside by a *yogī*, it is called *bahiḥ-kumbhaka* or *recita*. 31.

Note. When *prāṇa* and *apāna* are suspended, a prolonged state of equanimity supervenes, which is *bahiṣṭha-kumbhhaka* (HTK-38:69-72). 31.

व्याहृत्य[1] ग्रथितास्तारैर्गायत्रीं च शिरोयुताम् ।
संस्मरन् रेचयेत्[2] सूर्यं बहिर्वायुं निरोधयेत् ॥ ३२ ॥

1. व्याहृत्यो–J. 2. रेचयत्–J.

vyāhṛtya grathitās-tārair-gāyatrīṃ ca śiroyutām ।
saṃsmaran recayet sūryaṃ bahir-vāyuṃ nirodhayet ।32।

ध्यायेच्छून्यं निराभासं स्वान्तरे सर्वशून्यकः ।
द्विकराज[1]मतं चाथ दिङ्मात्रमिह वक्ष्यते ॥ ३३ ॥

dhyāyec-chūnyaṃ nirābhāsaṃ svāntare sarva-śūnyakaḥ ।
dvikarāja-mataṃ cātha diṅ-mātram-iha vakṣyate ॥ 33 ॥

Tr. When the air is exhaled through the right nostril while mentally repeating *gāyatrī* along with *praṇava (om)*, *vyāhṛti* and *śiras* and the breath is held outside, while contemplating on the internal void, it is *sarva-śūnyaka* according to *dvika-rāja (kāka)* told in a nut shell. 32-33.

Note. There are seven *vyāhṛtis* namely, *bhūḥ, bhuvaḥ, svaḥ, mahaḥ, janaḥ, tapaḥ* and *satyam*. The popular *mantra* in *gāyatrī* metre is –

tat savitur-vareṇyaṃ bhargo devasya dhīmahi ।
dhiyo yo naḥ pracodayāt ॥
praṇava is —*om*.
śiras is —
āpo jyoti raso'mṛtam brahma-bhūr-bhuvaḥ svarom ॥ 32-33.

पूरितोऽपानकुम्भः[2] स्याद् रेचितः प्राणकुम्भकः ।
रेचपूरौ तयोस्तद् द्विकराजमतं[3] त्विदम् ॥ ३४ ॥

pūrito'pāna-kumbhaḥ syād recitaḥ prāṇa-kumbhakaḥ ।
reca-pūrau tayos-tad dvikarāja-mataṃ tvidam ॥ 34 ॥

Tr. According to *dvika-rāja*, with inhaled air it is *apāna-kumbhaka*, while with exhaled air it is *prāṇa-kumbhaka*. They essentially comprise retention after exhalation and inhalation. 34.

Note. '*dvika*' means '*kāka*', there being two '*kas*' in the word. 34.

स्वतो हृत्खादुन्मुखता प्राणानायम्य यत्नतः[4] ।
आद्योऽयं बाह्यपूरो वा संज्ञायुग्मं तथान्यतः ॥ ३५ ॥

---

1. तद्विकराज–J. 2. कुम्भ–J. 3. मतं–not in J. 4. प्राणानामन्तरेचकः–**A**.

svato hṛt-khād-unmukhatā prāṇān-āyamya yatnataḥ ।
ādyo'yaṃ bāhya-pūro vā saṅjñā-yugmaṃ tathānyataḥ । 35।

Tr. The *prāṇa* which has natural tendency to rise upwards from the chest cavity, when controlled, is called *bāhya-pūraka*. The other two definitions are as follows: 35.

हृत्खान्तः सांगतो वायुः बाह्योऽन्यः प्राणपूरकः ॥ ३६ ॥

hṛt-khāntaḥ sāṅgato vāyuḥ bāhyo'nyaḥ prāṇa-pūrakaḥ ।36।

Tr. When the external *vāyu* enters the lungs to its limit, it is another variety of *bāhya-prāṇa-pūraka*. 36.

शरीरान्निर्गतिर्वायोर्द्वादशांगुलबाह्यखम् ।
बहिः प्राणस्य पूरोऽयं तृतीयः काकभाषितः ॥ ३७ ॥

śarīrān-nirgatir-vāyor-dvādaśāṅgula-bāhya-kham ।
bahiḥ prāṇasya pūro'yaṃ tṛtīyaḥ kākabhāṣitaḥ ॥ 37 ॥

Tr. According to *kāka*, when the *vāyu* comes out of the body and moves upto twelve digits (nine inches), it is the third kind of *bāhya-prāṇa-pūraka*. 37.

शरीरादुद्गतः प्राणो नासाग्राद् द्वादशांगुले ।
स्थिरो बहिःस्थे कुम्भः[1] स्याद्यावन्नापानसम्भवः[2] ॥ ३८ ॥

śarīrād-udgataḥ prāṇo
nāsāgrād dvādaśāṅgule ॥
sthiro bahiḥsthe kumbhaḥ syād-
yāvan-nāpāna-sambhavaḥ ॥ 38 ॥

Tr. When *prāṇa* moves out upto twelve digits (nine inches) from the tip of the nose while no further exhalation is possible, and when held outside, it is called *bahistha-kumbhaka*. 38.

Note. See note on KP-31. 38.

द्वादशांगुलखाद्वायुर्नासिकायां[3] तमिच्छति ।
आन्तरोऽपानपूरोऽयमाद्यश्चण्डात्मजोदितः ॥ ३९ ॥

---

1. कुम्भ–J. 2. स्याद् यावन्नो नासिकानुगः–A. 3. तु extra in J.

dvādaśāṅgula-khād-vāyur-nāsikāyāṃ tam-icchati ।
āntaro'pāna-pūro'yam-ādyaś-caṇḍātmajoditaḥ ॥ 39 ॥

Tr. According to *caṇḍātmaja*, when the *vāyu* moves into the nose from twelve digits outside, it is termed as the first variety of *āntara-apāna-pūraka*. 39.

बाह्यान्नासान्तमायाते द्वितीयोऽपानपूरकः ।
हृत्खं नासाग्रतो याति ह्यपाने पूरकोऽन्तिमः ॥
पूरितो हृद्यपानश्चेत् स्थिरो मृदि घटो यथा ॥ ४० ॥

bāhyān-nāsāntam-āyāte dvitīyo'pāna-pūrakaḥ ।
hṛt-khaṃ nāsāgrato yāti hyapāne pūrako'ntimaḥ ॥
pūrito hṛdyapānaś-cet sthiro mṛdi ghaṭo yathā ॥ 40 ॥

Tr. When it (*prāṇa*) enters into the end of the nose from outside, it is the second variety of *apāna-pūraka*.

Just as an earthen pot is a transformation of earth, similarly, when the air enters the chest from the tip of the nose, this is called *apāna-pūraka*, the last (third) variety. 40.

अपानेनोन्मुखः [1]वायुरन्तश्चान्द्रः स कुम्भकः ।
यस्मिंस्थितौ साक्षिमात्रे प्राणापानजयोदयौ ॥ ४१ ॥

apānenonmukhaḥ vāyur-
antaś-cāndraḥ sa kumbhakaḥ ॥
yasmiṅ-sthitau sākṣimātre
prāṇāpāna-jayodayau ॥ 41 ॥

Tr. Being stimulated by *apāna*, when *prāṇa-vāyu* moves upwards, it is called *cānrda-kumbhaka*. In this state, one experiences restraint of *prāṇa* and *apāna*. 41.

Note. By stimulation of *prāṇa* upwards with *apāna* here probably means application of *mūla-bandha*. 41.

सुखी स्यात् प्राणनियमे तत्तत्वस्यावधारणात् ।
प्राणापानकृता चेष्टा या हि यस्य[2] प्रवर्त्तते ॥ ४२ ॥

---

1. प्राण extra in J. 2. यस्या–J.

sukhī syāt prāṇa-niyame tat-tatvasyāvadhāraṇāt ।
prāṇāpāna-kṛtā ceṣṭā yā hi yasya pravartate ॥ 42 ॥

Tr. One becomes happy by meditating on *tatva* (Self) during *prāṇāyāma*, in which manipulation of *prāṇa* and *apāna* is involved. 42.

तच्चितेरनुसन्धानाज्जरामरणवर्जितः ।
सर्वसौभाग्यसहितः सर्वदुःखविवर्जितः ॥ ४३ ॥

tac-citer-anusandhānāj-jarā-maraṇa-varjitaḥ ।
sarva-saubhāgya-sahitaḥ sarva-duḥkha-vivarjitaḥ ॥ 43 ॥

Tr. By transcendental contemplation one becomes free from old age, premature death and all sufferings and attains all fortunes. 43.

Note. The word `*citi*' may also stand for funeral pyre on which concentration is suggested. 43.

भूतेन्द्रियप्रकृतिजित् सर्वज्ञः सर्वसिद्धियुक् ।
भुशुण्ड[1] इव दीर्घायुर्जायते नात्र संशयः [2] ॥ ४४ ॥

bhūtendriya-prakṛti-jit sarvajñaḥ sarva-siddhi-yuk ।
bhuśuṇḍa iva dīrghāyur-jāyate nātra saṅśayaḥ ॥ 44 ॥

Tr. When one attains control over senses and *prakṛti*, one becomes omniscient, attains all powers and lives long like *bhuśuṇḍa* in which there is no doubt. 44.

Note. In the *bṛhaj-jābālopaniṣad* we get a dialogue between *bhuśuṇḍa* and *kālāgni-rudra* describing various topics of *yogic* and ritualistic practices. In *rāmacaritamānasa* compossed by *santa tulasīdāsa*, we come across a reference to *bhuśuṇḍīrāmāyaṇa* authored by one *kākabhuśuṇḍī* who was a devotee of Lord *śrīrāma.* It is not known whether *kākabhuśuṇḍī* and *buśuṇḍa* are one and the same. 44.

संज्ञाज्ञानकृतो भेदः क्रियासु न भिदा स्फुटा ।
मूलशास्त्रादिति प्रोक्तं भुशुण्ड[1]मतमुत्तमम् ॥ ४५ ॥

---

1. भुसुण्ड–J. 2. शंशयः–J.

sañjñā-jñāna-kṛto bhedaḥ kriyāsu na bhidā sphuṭā ।
mūla-śāstrād-iti proktaṃ bhuśuṇḍa-matam-uttamam ॥45॥

Tr. According to the original tradition and also the opinion of *bhuśuṇḍa*, there is no apparent difference in the practice, although some difference may be found in the terms used. 45.

अथ वक्ष्ये दशविधप्राणानां निग्रहं परम् ॥ ४६ ॥

atha vakṣye daśa-vidha-prāṇānāṃ nigrahaṃ param ॥ 46 ॥

Tr. Now I shall describe the control of ten types of *prāṇa*. 46.

Note. The control of *prāṇa* extended to *pañca-prāṇas* (five *prāṇas*) and *pañca-upa-prāṇas* (five subordinate *prāṇas*) is seen only in this text. These ten-fold *prāṇas* are synonymously referred to as ten-fold *vāyus* in KP-83. These *prāṇas* or *vāyus* are reflexes forming the life-function. These may be stated as: - *prāṇa* (respiratory reflex that controls inhalation and exhalation), *apāna* (reflex governing excretory functions), *samāna* (reflex controlling the distribution of food and juices (fluids) through circulation), *vyāna* (reflex controlling cutaneous sensation), *udāna* (reflex controlling the movements of the body), *nāga* (reflex controlling hunger and thirst), *kūrma* (reflex controlling winking of eyes), *kṛkara* (sneezing reflex), *devadatta* (yawning reflex) and *dhanañjaya* (production of sound). YuB prescribes the technique of controlling the five *prāṇas* or *vāyus* by means of repeated inhalation and exhalation, concentration at the region of a particular *vāyu* and repeatetion of the respective *bīja*. For details see YuB-VII.54-78. 46.

प्राणो मुखघ्राणगतिराहृद्वृत्तिः समीरणः ।
गोनर्दीयमतं प्रोक्तमृषयोऽङ्गुष्ठके[1] पदे[2] ॥
नासाग्रनाभिहृत्संस्थं प्राहुस्तज्जय ईरितः ॥ ४७ ॥

prāṇo mukha-ghrāṇa-gatir-āhṛd-vṛttiḥ samīraṇaḥ ।
gonardīya-mataṃ proktam-ṛṣayo'ṅguṣṭhake pade ॥
nāsāgra-nābhi-hṛt-saṃsthaṃ prāhus-taj-jaya īritaḥ ॥ 47 ॥

1. ऽंगुष्टके–J. 2. पदो–J.

Tr. According to *gonardīya*, *prāṇa-vāyu* flows through mouth and nose upto the chest, while according to the *ṛṣis*, it is in the toes, tip of the nose, umbilicus and chest. Control of these *prāṇas* is indicated here. 47.

Note. The opinion of *gonardīya* about the region of *prāṇa* is stated here. The word *gonardīya* refers to the person coming from *gonarda* region which was the birthplace of *pātañjali* (author of *mahābhāṣya* on *aṣṭādhyāyī* of *pāṇini*). 47.

निःश्वासोच्छ्वासकर्मास्य तज्जये फलमीर्यते ।
विण्मूत्रश्लेष्मपित्तादिरोगदोषमनोमलाः ॥
सप्तधातुमला दोषा नश्यन्तीत्याह शंकरः ॥ ४८ ॥

niḥśvāsocchvāsa-karmāsya taj-jaye phalam-īryate ।
viṇ-mūtra-śleṣma-pittādi-roga-doṣa-mano-malāḥ ॥
sapta-dhātu-malā doṣā naśyantītyāha śaṅkaraḥ ॥ 48 ॥

Tr. Exhalation and inhalation are its functions. Their control leads to elimination of the impurities like faeces, urine, phlegm and bile which cause diseases of the body and also the mental impurities. According to *śaṅkara*, the impurities of the seven bodily constituents and (three) *doṣas* (humours like *vāta, pitta* and *kapha*) are removed. 48.

Note. According to *āyurveda*, the *sapta*- (seven) *dhātus* are the seven constituent elements of the body mentioned as chyle, blood, flesh, fat, bone, marrow and semen. *dhātu-mala* refers to the imbalance caused in one or more of these constituent elements. 48.

नादश्रुतिर्मेधा दीर्घमायुः[1] पुमर्थता ।
सुरूपता[2] बलं तेजः स्थिरता स्वरसौष्ठवम्[3] ॥ ४९ ॥

nādaśrutir-medhā dīrgham-āyuḥ pumarthatā ।
surūpatā balaṃ tejaḥ sthiratā svara-sauṣṭhavam ॥ 49 ॥

लघुत्वं शीघ्रगामित्वं कुण्डलीबोधनं परम् ।
उत्साहं च चिरोच्छ्वासं सुवर्णत्वादिकान् गुणान् ॥ ५० ॥

---

1. दीर्घसायुः–HSC. 2. स्वरूपता–HSC. 3. स्वरसौष्ठवः–HSC.

laghutvaṃ śīghra-gāmitvaṃ kuṇḍalī-bodhanaṃ param ।
utsāhaṃ ca cirocchvāsaṃ suvarṇatvādikān guṇān ॥ 50 ॥

सत्वस्थत्वं[1] च लभते योगी प्राणस्य निर्जये ।
भूचराणां जयः[2] सिध्येदित्याहुः शाम्भवा अपि[3] ॥ ५१ ॥

satvasthatvaṃ ca labhate yogī prāṇasya nirjaye ।
bhū-carāṇāṃ jayaḥ siddhyed-ityāhuḥ śāmbhavā api ॥ 51 ॥

Tr. Through the control of *prāṇa*, a *yogī* attains—hearing of mystical sounds, intelligence, long life, four aims of human existence, good look, strength, luster, stability, good voice, lightness, swiftness, arousal of *kuṇḍalinī*, enthusiasm, longer inhalation, a beautiful complexion and increase in *satva-guṇa*. According to *śāmbhavas*, one gains control over the living beings on the earth. 48-51.

Note. Four aims of human existence are *dharma, artha, kāma* and *mokṣa*. For evolution of *kuṇḍalinī* and its qualities, see SSP-I.7,12.

RY-35:6-168 gives 1008 names of *kuṇḍalinī* all beginning with *ka*. *śabda-brahma* is supposed to reside in *kuṇḍalinī*. 49-51.

आपादतलवृत्तिः स्यान्नाभेश्चाधोगतिः[4] स्वतः ॥ ५२ ॥[5]

āpādatala-vṛttiḥ syān-nābheś-cādhogatiḥ svataḥ ॥ 52 ॥

विण्मूत्रादिविसर्गं च कुरुतेऽपानसंज्ञितः ।
इति भाष्यमतं प्रोक्तमितरेषां[6] निगद्यते ॥ ५३ ॥

viṇ-mūtrādi-visargaṃ ca kurute'pāna-saṃjñitaḥ ।
iti bhāṣyamataṃ proktamitareṣāṃ nigadyate ॥ 53 ॥

Tr. One attains (proper) downward movement from navel to the feet facilitating excretion of urine and faeces which is the activity of *apāna*. This is narrated in the *bhāṣya*. Other opinions are narrated as follows: 52-53.

---

1. सत्वस्थलं–HSC. 2. चयः–HSC. 3. आह शशिशेखर इति–HSC. 4. गति–HSC.
5. अपान आपादतलैकवृत्तिरुदान आयस्तकवृत्तिरुच्चैः ।
आनाभिवृत्तिः समगो समानो व्यानस्तनौ व्याप्याभितोऽस्ति पुंसो ॥ –extra in HTK. 6. मितरेषा–J.

Note. *bhāṣya-mata* refers to the opinion of the commentator but the name of the commentator has not been suggested. 52-53.

कृकाटिकापृष्ठ[1]पार्ष्णिपृष्ठान्तेषु स्थितः शशी ।
रेचकाभ्यासबाहुल्यात्[2] क्रमात्स्थाननियोगतः ॥ ५४ ॥
kṛkāṭikā-pṛṣṭha-pārṣṇi-pṛṣṭhānteṣu sthitaḥ śaśī ।
recakābhyāsa-bāhulyāt kramāt-sthāna-niyogataḥ ॥ 54 ॥
ऊर्ध्वोर्ध्वमित्यपानस्य कुम्भकोर्ध्वजसंज्ञितः[3] ।
परकायप्रवेशः[4] स्याद् घटिकाद्वितयोन्मिते ॥ ५५ ॥
ūrddhvordhvamityapānasya kumbhakordhvajasaṃjñitaḥ ।
parakāya-praveśaḥ syād ghaṭikā-dvitayonmite ॥ 55 ॥

Tr. *śaśī* is situated in the neck, back, heel and the lower back. When one practises frequent *recakas* and by visualising concentrates on *apāna* from place to place, it is called *ūrdhvaja-kumbhaka*. Practice of this for two *ghaṭikās* (48 minutes) leads to *parakāya-praveśa siddhi* (ability to enter into another body). 54-55.

Note. The *yogic* literature refers to the location of *candra* or *śaśī* (moon) in the head (upper region) and not in the lower region. However, *nārāyaṇa tīrtha*, while commenting on `*viśokā vā jyotiṣmatī*' (YSC on PYS-I.36) refers to the location of *candra* below the heart region and the *sūrya-maṇḍala* (solar region). Thus, it somewhat corresponds to the location of *candra* in the lower region of the body as stated here. 54-55.

अपानं कटिदेशस्य[5] पृष्ठभागे विधारयेत् ।
सदा चेत् कुम्भकस्तज्जिन्मृग[6] इत्युच्यते बुधैः ॥ ५६ ॥
apānaṃ kaṭideśasya pṛṣṭha-bhāge vidhārayet ।
sadā cet kumbhakas-taj-jin-mṛga ityucyate budhaiḥ ॥ 56 ॥

Tr. According to the learned, when *apāna* is continuously held in the back of the hip region, it is known as *mṛga-kumbhaka*. 56.

---

1. पृष्ट–J. 2. बाहुल्या–HSC. 3. कुम्भकोध्वजसंज्ञिकः–J. 4. प्रवेशस्य–HSC. 5. कटिदेशेस्य–HSC. 6. कुम्भकस्तर्हिनिसर्ग–HSC.

मूलबन्धो धारणासु मुद्राविषयगोचरः ।
गूथ[1]मूत्राल्पता वह्नेर्जाठरस्य प्रदीपनम् ॥ ५७ ॥
mūla-bandho dhāraṇāsu mudrā-viṣaya-gocaraḥ ।
gūtha-mūtrālpatā vahner-jāṭharasya pradīpanam ॥ 57 ॥
कुण्डलीबोधनं चैव ब्रह्मरन्ध्रप्रवेशनम् ।
पातालगमनं चैव लीलया जायते मुनेः ॥ ५८ ॥
kuṇḍalī-bodhanaṃ caiva brahmarandhra-praveśanam ।
pātāla-gamanaṃ caiva līlayā jāyate muneḥ ॥ 58 ॥
क्षतस्य रोहणं स्वात्म्यं बहुभोजनरूग्जयौ ।
सत्वात्मकत्वं स्युश्चान्येऽप्यपानस्य जये गुणाः ॥ ५९ ॥
kṣatasya rohaṇaṃ svātmyaṃ bahubhojana-rug-jayau ।
satvātmakatvaṃ syuś-cānye'pyapānasya jaye guṇāḥ ॥59॥

Tr. The benefits of control of *apāna* are facilitation of *mūlabandha*, proficiency in the practice of *dhāraṇā* and different *mudrās*, reduction in urine and faeces, increase in gastric fire, arousal of *kuṇḍalinī* and its entry into *brahma-randhra, pātāla-gamana* (traveling to the world underneath), healing of the wounds, assimilation of all food, conquest of all diseases and increase in *satva-guṇa* etc. 57-59.

Note. In *haṭha-yogic* literarure, *mūlābandha* is included under the *mudrās* (see HP(L)-IV.6, GhS-III.13 etc.). GhS-III.2 includes five *dhāraṇās* under the *mudrās.*

For details on *dhāraṇā*, see HP(L)-VI.10-18. According to HP(L)-V.6-7, there are ten *mudrās,* while JP-512-727 puts the number of *mudrās* to 24. See HP(L)-V.6-7. 57-59.

आनाभिहृदयाद् भाष्ये समानस्थानमीरितम् ।
सर्वसन्धिस्थितोऽपीति प्राहुरन्ये महर्षयः ॥ ६० ॥
ānābhi-hṛdayād bhāṣye samāna-sthānam-īritam ।
sarva-sandhi-sthito'pīti prāhur-anye maharṣayaḥ ॥ 60 ॥

Tr. The location of *samāna-vāyu* is stated to be in the region from navel to the chest. Other authorities maintain that it exists in all the joints. 60.

---

1. गूप्य–J.

Note. About the region of *samāna*, two opinions have been mentioned. i) From navel to the heart, ii) all the joints. However, we find texts like VS-II.48 mentioning the region of *samāna* in the whole body. 60.

समं रसानां[1] नयनं[2] कर्मास्य परिकीर्त्तितम् ॥ ६१ ॥

samaṃ rasānāṃ nayanaṃ karmāsya parikīrtitam ॥ 61 ॥

Tr. Its function is said to be proper distribution of nutrition (bodily fluids). 61.

नाभावापूर्य वायु[3]श्चेद्देहे व्याप्य विधारितः ।
कुम्भिते[4] ज्वलनं ध्यायेत्[5] समानस्य तु कुम्भकः ॥ ६२ ॥

nābhāvāpūrya vāyuś-ced-dehe vyāpya vidhāritaḥ ।
kumbhite jvalanaṃ dhyāyet samānasya tu kumbhakaḥ ।62।

Tr. When this *vāyu* is filled up into the navel and held with concentration on fire, it is *samāna-kumbhaka*. 62.

[6]मुद्रासु वक्ष्यते कुम्भ उड्डियानो महाफलः ।
एजते[7] प्रज्वलेत्[8] स्विद्ये[9]द्रोमकूपेषु मोचयेत्[10] ॥
तमेव व्यापकं योगी सोऽयं नकुलीशमतं तथा[11] ॥ ६३ ॥

mudrāsu vakṣyate kumbha uḍḍiyāno mahāphalaḥ ।
ejate prajvalet svidyed-roma-kūpeṣu mocayet ॥
*tam-eva vyāpakaṃ yogī so'yaṃ nakulīśa-mataṃ tathā*63

Tr. This practice is recommended in *mudrās*, as it results in attaining *uḍḍiyāna*. This is explained in terms of movement, heat, perspiration and sensation in the pores extensively experienced by a *yogī*. This is the opinion of *nakulīśa*. 63.

---

1. समरसानाम्-HTK. 2. नय-HTK. 3. नाभौ पूर्यसमीरं –HTK, HSC. 4. कुभिते-HTK, कुम्भिके-HSC. 5. ध्याये -HSC. 6. line not in A. 7. राधते-HTK. 8. प्रज्वलन् –HTK. 9. खिद्येत् –HSC. 10. योजयेत्–HSC,HTK. 11. नकुलो शमनं तथा–HSC, प्रज्वालनो मतः–J.

क्षुत्तृट्क्षयो वह्निदीप्तिः क्षतभग्नावरोहणम् ।
समानकुम्भकाभ्यासात् फलं स्यादिति शंकरः ॥ ६४ ॥[1]

kṣut-tṛṭ-kṣayo vahni-dīptiḥ kṣata-bhagnāvarohaṇam ।
samāna-kumbhakābhyāsāt phalaṃ syād-iti śaṅkaraḥ ।64।

Tr. The results of *samāna-kumbhaka* maintained by *śaṅkara* are control of hunger and thirst, increased gastric fire, (quick) healing of wounds and fractures. 64.

व्यानो व्यापी व्यानयनस्त्वगिन्द्रियनिकेतनः ॥ ६५ ॥

vyāno vyāpī vyānayanas-tvag-indriya-niketanaḥ ॥ 65 ॥

Tr. The *vyāna* pervades all over the body and sense organs like skin etc. 65.

पूरयित्वान्तरा सम्यग् हृज्जगद्व्याप्तियोगतः ।
सर्वांगस्याकुञ्चनेन[2] कुम्भिते सूक्ष्मचिन्तनात् ॥
पार्वतीवक्त्रभेनोक्तः सम्यक् व्यानस्य कुम्भकः ॥ ६६ ॥

pūrayitvāntarā samyag hṛj-jagad-vyāpti-yogataḥ ।
sarvāṅgasyākuñcanena kumbhite sūkṣma-cintanāt ॥
pārvatī-vaktrabhenoktaḥ samyak vyānasya kumbhakaḥ 66।

Tr. *vyāna-kumbhaka* is described by *pārvatī* as completely filling the chest and contracting the whole body during *kumbhaka* with subtle concentration. 66.

न शस्त्रैश्छिद्यते नापः क्लेदयन्त्यविषक्रमः[3] ।
शीतोष्णयोस्तथासंगो[4] रोगनाशश्च जायते[5] ॥ ६७ ॥

na śastraiś-chidyate nāpaḥ kledayantyaviṣa-kramaḥ ।
śītoṣṇayos-tathāsaṅgo roga-nāśaś-ca jāyate ॥ 67 ॥

Tr. (The results of *vyāna-kumbhaka* are described in terms of) protection from weapons, water and poisons, immunity from cold and heat and removal of diseases. 67.

---

1. Verse not in A. 2. सर्वांगमाकुञ्चनेन –HTK. 3. अपि विषयक्रमः -HSC. 4. शीतोष्णस्त्वचासंगो –A. 5. रोगनाशस्त्रैः छिद्यते –HTK.

उदान उन्नयनाकवृत्तिर्भाष्य उदाहृतः ।
घण्टिकामध्यताल्वग्रपतलेष्विति[1] चापरे ॥ ६८ ॥

udāna unnayanāka-vṛttir-bhāṣya udāhṛtaḥ ।
ghaṇṭikā-madhya-tālvagra-pataleṣviti cāpare ॥ 68 ॥

Tr. As narrated in the commentaries, *udāna* means that which rises up. Its location is described by some in uvula, mid-palate and tips of the tongue. 68.

Note. The region of *udāna* is stated to be uvula, mid-palate and tip of the tongue, which according to other authorities like VS-II.47 and others is in all the joints.

The sequence of the five *prāṇas* is not the same given in different *yogic* texts. The GŚ-V.60 and VāPu-XV.7-8 mention the *vāyus* in the same sequence as given by VS-II.42 which is *prāṇa, apāna, samāna, udāna* and *vyāna.* But ChU-III.13, V.19-23, MhB-184.24-25 and BYS follow a different order as *prāṇa, vyāna, apāna, samāna* and *udāna*. In BrA-III.9-26 the sequence is *prāṇa, apāna, vyāna, udāna* and *samāna* which is widely accepted. TtA-X.33.1-5 mentions the *vāyus* as *prāṇa, apāna, udāna, samāna* and *udāna*. VB follows the different sequence as *prāṇa, samāna* , *apāna, udāna* and *vyāna.* For this difference in the sequence of the *vāyus* no adequate explanation can be given. 68.

नोभ्यां चाकर्षयेद्वायुं[2] बलात् हृत्स्थानमानयेत् ।
उत्कृष्योत्कृष्य हृत्स्थानात् कण्ठतालौ[3] भ्रुवोऽन्तरे[4] ॥
मूर्ध्नान्तं[5] चेदगतायातकृत्ति[6]श्रेष्ठाख्यकुम्भकः[7] ॥ ६९ ॥

nobhyāṃ cākarṣayed-vāyuṃ balāt hṛt-sthānam-ānayet ।
utkṛṣyotkṛṣya hṛt-sthānāt kaṇṭha-tālau bhruvo'ntare ॥
mūrdhnāntaṃ ced-gatāyāta-kṛtti-śreṣṭhākhya-kumbhakaḥ ।69।

1. पत्तलेष्विति –A. 2. नासाभ्यां कर्षयेद् –HTK. 3. कण्ठे -HTK, HSC. 4. भ्रुवोन्तरे –HSC. 5. मूर्धानं –HSC. 6. गतापानकृतिः -HSC. 7. रतायतकृतिश्चेष्टाख्य-J. 8. मूर्धान्तं चेद् गतायातकृत्तिश्चेष्टाख्यकुम्भकः -A.

Tr. One should forcibly raise the *vāyu* bringing it into chest through nostrils and from there take it further to the throat, palate, mid-brow, top of the head and retain it there. This is *kṛtti-śreṣtha-kumbhaka*. 69.

वान्वितेनाशुगं[1] कर्षेन्[2] कुर्वन्तूच्चतरं स्वनम्[3] ।
धारयेच्चेदुदानस्य प्रकृतिः[4] कुम्भकः स्मृतः ॥ ७० ॥

vānvitenāśugaṃ karṣen kurvantūccataraṃ svanam ।
dhārayec-ced-udānasya prakṛtiḥ kumbhakaḥ smṛtaḥ ॥70॥

Tr. Sucking the air with a loud sound with *(bīja-mantra)* '*va*' and holding it is known as *prakṛti-kumbhaka*. 70.

जले पंके कण्टकेषु न संगः[5] स्यात्कदाचन ।
खगत्वमुत्क्रान्तिरपीत्येतत् फलमुदाहृतम् ॥ ७१ ॥

jale paṅke kaṇṭakeṣu na saṅgaḥ syāt-kadācana ।
khagatvam-utkrāntir-apītyetat phalam-udāhṛtam ॥ 71 ॥

Tr. The results of this *kumbhaka* are mentioned in terms of remaining ever unaffected by water, mud and thorns and also attaining ability to levitate. 71.

स्वस्वस्थानात् समाकृष्य पिण्डीकृत्य हृदम्बुजे ।
वह्नींश्च ब्रह्मरन्ध्रान्तः नमनात् सर्वजिद् भवेत् ॥ ७२ ॥

sva-sva-sthānāt samākṛṣya
piṇḍīkṛtya hṛd-ambuje ॥
vahnīṅś-ca brahmarandhrāntaḥ
namanāt sarvajid bhavet ॥ 72 ॥

Tr. By taking *vahni (kuṇḍalinī* along with *prāṇa)* from respective places, condensing it in the lotus of the heart and uniting into *brahma-randhra*, one gains control over all the *vāyus*. 72.

---

1. नाशुगः -HTK, कान्वितेनाशुगं –J. 2. कर्षन् –HTK, HSC. 3. कुञ्च्य कुञ्च्यतरं स्वनं –HSC. 4. प्राहूतिः -HTK, पदगति –A. 5. संगे –HSC.

सर्वमेव फलं भूयाद्वायूनां युगपज्जये ।
रेचकाभ्यासतः सर्ववायूनां युगपज्जयः ॥ ७३ ॥

sarvam-eva phalaṃ bhūyād-vāyūnāṃ yugapaj-jaye ।
recakābhyāsataḥ sarva-vāyūnāṃ yugapaj-jayaḥ ॥ 73 ॥

Tr. By the practice of *recaka* (control on exhalation) one also controls all the *vāyus*. By controlling the *vāyus* one simultaneously gets all the results. 73.

नीत्वा वायुं नाभिमध्यं सूर्याग्रे योऽस्य रेचनात् ।
सर्ववायुजयो भूयादित्याहुर्मुनयः परे ॥ ७४ ॥

nītvā vāyuṃ nābhi-madhyaṃ sūryāgre yo'sya recanāt ।
sarva-vāyujayo bhūyād-ityāhur-munayaḥ pare ॥ 74 ॥

Tr. By moving the *vāyu* in the center of the navel and exhalaing the same through the *sūrya-nāḍī* (right nostril), one attains control of all the *vāyus* (*prāṇas*) as stated by some *munis*. 74.

अतः समाधेरभ्यासादपि सर्वजयो भवेत् ॥ ७५ ॥

ataḥ samādher-abhyāsād-api sarva-jayo bhavet ॥ 75 ॥

Tr. By the practice of *samādhi* also one controls all the *vāyus* (*prāṇas*). 75.

सुषुम्णा ग्रसते तस्मिन् यतो वायुपरम्पराम् ।
अशेषकल्पनानाशः पूर्वोक्तं च फलं भवेत् ॥ ७६ ॥

suṣumṇā grasate tasmin yato vāyu-paramparām ।
aśeṣa-kalpanā-nāśaḥ pūrvoktaṃ ca phalaṃ bhavet ॥ 76 ॥

Tr. When *prāṇa* is controlled, the *vāyus* enter *suṣumṇā* resulting into disappearance of all the thoughts and attaining all the results stated above. 76.

Note. HP also refers to the same process when it says that as *prāṇa* moves through *suṣumṇā* and *manas* (mind) merges into the void, the *yogī* is no longer bound by the law of *karma* (action) and the state of `*manonmanī*' is achieved (HP(L)-V.78,VII.30,VIII.50). 76.

ओदन[1]ग्रासवद्वायुं कण्ठेनापूरयेच्छनैः ।
तं रोधयेद्यथाकालं बध्वा जालन्धरं दृढम् ॥ ७७ ॥

odana-grāsavad-vāyuṃ kaṇṭhenāpūrayec-chanaiḥ ।
taṃ rodhayed-yathākālaṃ badhvā jālandharaṃ dṛḍham ।77।

कण्ठेन रेचनं कुर्यान्नागकुम्भः शिवोदितः ।
क्षुधां[2] जयेत् पिपासां च फलमस्य समीरितम् ॥ ७८ ॥

kaṇṭhena recanaṃ kuryān-nāga-kumbhaḥ śivoditaḥ ।
kṣudhāṃ jayet pipāsāṃ ca phalam-asya samīritam ॥ 78 ॥

Tr. One should swallow the air slowly into the throat like a morsel of rice, retaining it to the capacity, with firm application of *jālandhara-bandha* and then expell it from the throat. This is *nāga-kumbhaka* explained by *śiva*. By this practice one is able to control hunger and thirst. 77-78.

Note. HR-II.32 gives a similar technique under the name of *bhujaṅgī-karaṇa* as one of the nine *kumbhakas*.

The technique of swallowing the air is described as *bhujaṅgī-mudrā* in GhS-III.69-70.

In *plāvinī-kumbhaka* also, the air is swallowed to fill the stomach as described in HP(L)-II.70.

While enumerating eight *kumbhakas*, HP(L)-IV.33 omits *plāvinī* and includes *kevala-kumbhaka*. GhS-V.46 omits *sītkārī* and *plāvinī* and substitutes *sahita* and *kevala*. 77-78.

निमीलोन्मीलने त्यक्त्वा पीठे काष्ठमिव स्थितिः[3] ।
नेत्रयोश्च शरीरस्य कूर्मकुम्भः[4] स उच्यते ॥
भवतोऽभ्यासवशान्मनोवातौ स्थिरावुभौ ॥ ७९ ॥

nimīlonmīlane tyaktvā pīṭhe kāṣṭham-iva sthitiḥ ।
netrayoś-ca śarīrasya kūrma-kumbhaḥ sa ucyate ॥
bhavato'bhyāsa-vaśān-mano-vātau sthirāvubhau ॥ 79 ॥

---

1. उदान-HTK. 2. क्षुधा-J.
3. निमीलोन्मीलनके विहाय स्थितिर्दृढकाष्ठमिवाप्राचाल्यादृशोस्तनोर्भुरि स कूर्मकुम्भः स्थैर्य करोत्याशुगचित्तयोर्हि-extra in HTK.
4. कूर्मकुम्भ -J.

Tr. When the blinking of the eyes is controlled and one becomes perfectely steady in an *āsana* like a log of wood and devoid of movements of the eyes and the body, it is called *kūrma-kumbhaka*. With the practice of this *kumbhaka*, one attains steadiness of *vāyu* and mind. 79.

Note. HSC calls *kūrma-kumbhaka* by another name as *trāṭaka*. Different texts also talk about *trāṭaka-kumbhaka* (JP-491-493, BB, SD etc.). HTK describes this process as control of *nāga-vāyu* but it does not mention about expelling of air from the throat. 79.

तर्जन्यनामिकेंऽगुष्ठमर्द्दिते क्षुतसम्भवे ।
क्षुतसंहरणः कुम्भः कृकरस्य जयप्रदः ॥ ८० ॥

tarjanyanāmike'ṅguṣṭha-marddite kṣuta-sambhave ।
kṣuta-saṃharaṇaḥ kumbhaḥ kṛkarasya jaya-pradaḥ ॥ 80 ॥

Tr. When there is a possibility of sneezing, one should rub index and ring fingers with the thumb. This controls sneeze and is known as *kṛkara-kumbhaka*. 80.

Note. It is interesting to note the technique of controlling sneeze, which is the function of *kṛkara-vāyu* by rubbing the index and ring fingers with the thumb. This obviously does not include the process of *kumbhaka*.

The author of HSC calls this as *avadhūta-jaya-prakriyā*. 80.

जृम्भोद्‌भवे संवृत्यास्यः[1] कण्ठाधः प्रापयेत्खगम् ।
देवदत्तजयस्तेन जायते शंकरोदितः ॥ ८१ ॥

jṛmbhodbhave saṃvṛtyāsyaḥ
kaṇṭhādhaḥ prāpayet-khagam ॥
devadatta-jayas-tena
jāyate śaṅkaroditaḥ ॥ 81 ॥

Tr. When yawning occurs, one should close the mouth and push the air down the throat. Accoding to *śaṅkara*, this leads to control of *deva-datta-vāyu*. 81.

---

1. संवृतास्यः -HTK.

देहस्थ[1]मखिलं वायुं कुण्डली ग्रसते यदा ।
धनञ्जयजयः काले तस्मिन् गौणस्ततो[2] ह्ययम्[3] ॥ ८२ ॥

dehastham-akhilaṃ vāyuṃ kuṇḍalī grasate yadā ।
dhanañjaya-jayaḥ kāle tasmin gauṇas-tato hyayam ॥ 82 ॥

Tr. When *kuṇḍalī* absorbs all the *vāyus* in the body, it is the control of *dhanañjaya-vāyu.* In this state everything becomes insignificant. 82.

इत्युक्तं दशवायूनां[4] जयोऽयं क्रमतो मया ।
पूर्वोक्ताभ्यासयोगेन युगपद्वा जयो भवेत् ॥ ८३ ॥

ityuktaṃ daśa-vāyūnāṃ jayo'yaṃ kramato mayā ।
pūrvoktābhyāsa-yogena yugapad-vā jayo bhavet ॥ 83 ॥

Tr. I have narrated control of ten *vāyus* progressively. With the practice as stated earlier, one attains complete mastery over them. 83.

Note. It will be found from the description given above that the control of ten *vāyus* or *prāṇas* is considered as *kumbhakas.* There is no retention of breath in controlling of the *prāṇas* like *kūrma* (KP-79), *kṛkara* (KP-80), *devadatta* (KP-81) and *dhanañjaya* (KP-82). 83.

हंसवेधं विना नैते सिध्यन्ति यमिनां क्वचित् ।
प्रत्युतानुभवत्येव रोगराशिं पदे पदे ॥
तस्मात् सुदीक्षितो योगी पवनाभ्यासमाचरेत् ॥ ८४ ॥[5]

haṃsavedhaṃ vinā naite siddhyanti yamināṃ kvacit ।
pratyutānubhavatyeva rogarāśiṃ pade pade ॥
tasmāt sudīkṣito yogī pavanābhyāsam-ācaret ॥ 84 ॥

Tr. These cannot be accomplished by the *yogī* without *haṃsa-vedha.* Otherwise, one has to face several diseases frequently. Therefore, a *yogī* should undertake the practice of *prāṇāyāma* only after receiveing proper instructions (initiation). 84.

---

1. देवस्थं-J. 2. तत-J. 3. हृदयं-HTK. 4. वायुनां –J. 5. Verse not in A.

Note. In spite of great importance given to the technique of *haṃsa-vedha,* it is nowhere described in the whole text (see note on KP-179). 84.

पूररेचयुतः कुम्भो वायोर्यत्र विधीयते ।
सहितः कुम्भकः स स्यात् सहितः सर्वसिद्धये ॥ ८५ ॥

pūra-reca-yutaḥ kumbho vāyor-yatra vidhīyate ।
sahitaḥ kumbhakaḥ sa syāt sahitaḥ sarva-siddhaye ॥ 85 ॥

Tr. When *vāyu* is restrained with *pūraka, kumbhaka* and *recaka*, it is *sahita-kumbhaka*, which brings all the benefits. 85.

सहितं कुम्भकं कुर्वन्नाडीशुद्धिं च विन्दति ।
केवलं कुम्भकं नादश्रवणं सिद्धयोऽखिलाः ॥ ८६ ॥

sahitaṃ kumbhakaṃ kurvan-nāḍī-śuddhiṃ ca vindati ।
kevalaṃ kumbhakaṃ nāda-śravaṇaṃ siddhayo'khilāḥ ।86।

Tr. *sahita-kumbhaka* brings purification of all the *nāḍīs*, while *kevala-kumbhaka* leads to hearing of mystical sounds and bestows all the supernatural powers. 86.

Note. According to GhS-V.47-58, *sahita-prāṇāyāma* forms one of the eight *kumbhakas,* which is two-fold: *sagarbha* and *nigarbha. sagarbha* is performed with *bīja* while *nigarbha* is practised without *bīja.* According to HTK-44:57, giving up *recaka* and *pūraka* all the time, the state of *kumbhaka* maintained naturally all the time is known as *kevala-kumbhaka.* Also see HTK-38:51, HP(L)-IV.63 for more details on *agarbha-sagarbha-prāṇāyāma.*

HP(L)-IV.63 sugests that *sahita-kumbhaka* should be practised until *kevala-kumbhaka* supervenes.

The *kumbhaka* that is accompanied by *pūraka* and *recaka* is called *sahita*, while *kumbhaka* irrespective of *pūraka* and *recaka* is called *kevala.* According to *devala,* there are seven types of *kumbhakas,* namely— *recita, pūrita, śānta, pratyāhāra, uttara, adhara* and *sama.* Out of these, *śānta* and *sama* fall under the category of *kevala-kumbhaka.* Under *sahita-kumbhaka* fall *pūrita, recita, uttara* and *adhara,* while *pratyāhāra* falls under both the categories.

The result of *sahita-kumbhaka* has been stated to be the purification of the *nāḍīs*, while *kevala-kumbhaka* leads to experience of mystical sound and success in *yoga*. *sahita-kumbhaka* leads to the attainment of *kevala-kumbhaka*. Thus *sahita-kumbhaka* is voluntary and *kevala-kumbhaka* is involuntary. 85-86.

सूर्येण पूरयेत् प्राणं कुम्भयित्वा यथाविधिः ।
रेचयेदन्यमार्गेण पुनस्तेन प्रपूरयेत् ॥
येन त्यजेत्तेनापूर्य चाग्निषोमाख्यकुम्भकः ॥ ८७ ॥

sūryeṇa pūrayet prāṇam kumbhayitvā yathā-vidhiḥ ।
recayed-anya-mārgeṇa punas-tena prapūrayet ॥
yena tyajet-tenāpūrya cāgni-ṣomākhya-kumbhakaḥ ॥ 87 ॥

Tr. *prāṇa* should be inhaled through *sūrya-nāḍī* (right-nostril) and after retaining the same as prescribed, one should exhale through the other nostril, and again inhale by the same side through which one has exhaled. It is known as *agni-ṣoma-kumbhaka*. 87.

Note. There seems to be some similarity of this practice with *anuloma-viloma* or *nāḍī-śodhaka-prāṇāyāma* (HP(L)-IV.11-15, GhS-V.38-45), except that in *anuloma-viloma* one starts inhaling through the left nostril, while in *agni-ṣoma* one starts inhaling through the right nostril. 87.

केवलं कुम्भयेत् प्राणं रेचपूरणवर्जितम् ।
तूर्यः शेषोदितोऽन्ये तु केवलं कुम्भकं विदुः ॥ ८८ ॥

kevalaṃ kumbhayet prāṇaṃ reca-pūraṇa-varjitam ।
tūryaḥ śeṣodito'nye tu kevalaṃ kumbhakaṃ viduḥ ॥ 88 ॥

Tr. *prāṇa* should be retained irrespective of inspiration or expiration. This is fourth variety of *kumbhaka*, called *kevala* by others. 88.

Note. The fourth variety of *prāṇāyāma* seems to refer to *patañjali's caturtha-prāṇāyāma* (PYS-II.51). 88.

मनोजवत्वं च मनोजयश्च
पालित्यहानिर्वलितस्य नाशः ॥

नादश्रुतिश्चाष्टविधास्य सिद्धिर्[1]
वायोर्जयः केवलकुम्भकात् स्यात् ॥ ८९ ॥

mano-javatvaṃ ca mano-jayaś-ca
pālitya-hānir-valitasya nāśaḥ ॥
nāda-śrutiś-cāṣṭavidhāsya siddhir-
vāyor-jayaḥ kevala-kumbhakāt syāt ॥ 89 ॥

Tr. Benefits of *kevala-kumbhaka* are stated as increased dexterity of mind, control of mental activities, disappearance of grey hair and wrinkles, hearing of mystical sounds, accomplishment of eight-fold *siddhis* and control of *vāyu*. 89.

कायस्यान्तर्बहिर्व्याप्तिः शान्तकुम्भक उदाहृतः ।
स्थानयोरन्तरे रुध्वा कुम्भयेद्यदि मारुतम् ॥ ९० ॥

kāyasyāntar-bahir-vyāptiḥ śānta-kumbhaka udāhṛtaḥ ।
sthānayor-antare ruddhvā kumbhayed-yadi mārutam ॥90॥

Tr. Restraining the *vāyu* inside and visualising its presence inside and outside of the body is called *śānta-kumbhaka*. 90.

नवस्थानानि विज्ञाय प्रत्याहारः स वेधसः ।
पादतलगुह्यनाभिहृदयोरःकण्ठघण्टिकाः क्रमतः ॥ ९१ ॥

nava-sthānāni vijñāya pratyāhāraḥ sa vedhasaḥ ।
pādatala-guhya-nābhi-hṛdayoraḥ-kaṇṭha-ghaṇṭikāḥ kramataḥ ॥ 91॥

भ्रूमध्यं च ललाटं ब्रह्मस्थानं नवैतानि ।
योगसिद्धिः सर्वरोगनाशः प्रत्याहृतौ भवेत् ॥ ९२ ॥

bhrū-madhyaṃ ca lalāṭaṃ brahmasthānaṃ navaitāni ॥
yogasiddhiḥ sarvaroga-nāśaḥ pratyāhṛtau bhavet ॥ 92 ॥

Tr. Soles, organs of generation, navel, heart, throat, uvula, middle of the eyebrows, forehead and *brahma-randhra* are the nine sites according to *vedhā (śiva)*. Concentration of *prāṇa* on one site and then another in this sequence is called *pratyāhāra*, which brings success in *yoga* and removes all diseases. 91-92.

---

1. सिद्धि-J.

Note. The nine sites mentioned by GP-II.75 are anus, organ of generation, navel, heart, the place above the heart, uvula, tongue, center of the eyebrows and *brahma-randhra* (*nabhobila*—crown of the head). In SSP-I.1-9 the *nava-sthānas* (nine sites) are described in the form of nine *cakras*, which are *brahma-cakra* in *mūlādhāra, svādhiṣṭhāna, nābhi-cakra, hṛdaya, kaṇṭha tālu, bhrū, brahma-randhra* and *ākāśa-cakra*. 91-92.

स्थानात् स्थानं समाकृष्य यदष्टदशकेष्वपि ।
ऋषिप्रोक्तः स कुम्भः स्यात् प्रत्याहारस्तु कुम्भनात् ॥ ९३ ॥

sthānāt sthānaṃ samākṛṣya yad-aṣṭa-daśakeṣvapi ।
ṛṣi-proktaḥ sa kumbhaḥ syāt pratyāhāras-tu kumbhanāt ।93।

Tr. Withdrawing *prāṇa* from all the eighteen vital points, one after another in sequence (during *kumbhaka*), becomes *ṛṣi-prokta-kumbhaka*. This process of *kumbhaka* is *pratyāhāra*. 93.

पादांगुष्ठो गुल्फो जंघामूलं चितेर्मूलम् ।
मध्यं जान्वोरुरुपायोर्मूलं स्वदेहमध्यं च ॥ ९४ ॥

pādāṅguṣṭho gulpho jaṅghā-mūlaṃ citer-mūlam ।
madhyaṃ jānvor-urupāyor-mūlaṃ svadeha-madhyaṃ ca ।94।

लिंगनाभिहृदयं कण्ठाधस्ता[1]लुमूलं च ।
घोणामूलं नयने भ्रूमध्यं वज्रकन्दकम्[2] ॥ ९५ ॥

liṅga-nābhi-hṛdayaṃ kaṇṭhādhas-tālu-mūlaṃ ca ।
ghoṇā-mūlaṃ nayane bhrū-madhyaṃ vajra-kandakam ।95।

Tr. (The eighteen vital points are as follows—) toes, ankle, root of the thigh, front part or the head of tibia, center of the knee, thigh, anus, center of the body, generative organ, navel, heart, root of the throat, root of the palate, root of the nose, eyes, middle of the eyebrows and *vajra-kanda* (*sahasrāra*). 94-95.

Note. In the list of eighteen vital points, one point between the center of the eyebrows and *vajra-kandaka* (=*sahasrāra*) seems to be missing. On the basis of the description of eighteen vital

1. कण्ठाधुस्-J. 2. वज्रकन्दःकं –J.

points in VS-III.61-64 this missing vital point may be considered as the forehead (*lalāṭa*). 94-95.

अष्टादशधा मुनयो वदन्ति दिव्यौ भिषग्वरौ दस्त्रौ ।
षोडश पातञ्जलिकाः षड्विंशच्छम्भुना प्रोक्ताः ॥ ९६ ॥

aṣṭādaśadhā munayo vadanti
divyau bhiṣag-varau dastrau ॥
ṣoḍaśa pātañjalikāḥ
ṣaḍ-viṃśac-chambhunā proktāḥ ॥ 96 ॥

Tr. The vital points are eighteen according to *munis* and the (two) *aśvinīkumāras*, the physicians of gods, sixteen according to the followers of *patañjali* and twenty-six according to *śambhu*. 96.

Note. According to Hindu mythology, *aśvinī-kumāras* are divine physicians.

There is no uniformity of the sites and number of the vital points. These sites are variously referred to in different texts as *sthāna*, *ādhāra* or *marma*. Different authorities differ in the description of these points, as stated also in this verse. According to *āyurveda*, *marmas* are vital points in the body hurting of which may cause death-like condition or even death (CS(sūtra)-11.48). According to SuS(śārīra)-VI.15, there are 107 *marma-sthānas* in the human body. 96.

[1]एतत् सकलं ज्ञेयं शरीरेषु गुरोरग्रे ।
क्रमतो व्युत्क्रमतोऽपि प्रत्याहारो भवेदेषु ॥ ९७ ॥

etat sakalaṃ jñeyaṃ śarīreṣu guror-agre ।
kramato vyut-kramato'pi pratyāhāro bhaved-eṣu ॥ 97 ॥

Tr. Knowing all these in the body from a *guru*, one should practise *pratyāhāra* in inverse and reverse orders. 97.

आपूर्योर्ध्वोर्ध्वं यो रोधो हृदादिषु स उत्तरः ।
मूर्ध्वतोऽधोऽध अधरो मुनिभिः परिभाषितः ॥ ९८ ॥

---

1. एवं मतान्तराण्यपि विस्तारभीत्या न लिख्यते –extra in A.

āpūryordhvordhvaṃ yo rodho hṛdādiṣu sa uttaraḥ ।
mūrdhvato'dho'dha adharo munibhiḥ paribhāṣitaḥ ॥ 98 ॥

Tr. Inhaling and holding (of *prāṇa*) from heart upwards (upto the top of the head) is called *uttara*, and from top of the head downwards upto the heart, is called *adhara* by the *munis*. 98.

आरेकपूरा[1] मनसा नाभ्यादाशुगं धृतिः ।
समः कुम्भो भगवता प्रोक्तः श्रीचन्द्रमौलिना ॥ ९९ ॥

ārekapūrā manasā nābhyād-āśugaṃ dhṛtiḥ ।
samaḥ kumbho bhagavatā proktaḥ śrī-candra-maulinā ।99।

Tr. Without actually inhaling or exhaling, when one mentally holds the *prāṇa* in the regions like navel etc., it is described as *sama-kumbhaka* by *bhagavān candra-mauli (śiva)*. 99.

यावन्निरोधसामर्थ्यं कर्षकः[2] कुम्भको द्विधा ॥ १०० ॥

yāvan-nirodha-sāmarthyaṃ karṣakaḥ kumbhako dvidhā ।100।

Tr. According to the capacity of retention, *karṣaka-kumbhaka* is two-fold. 100.

नासामूलं मुद्रयित्वा तदग्रे रेचपूरकौ ।
कुर्यादुत्कर्षकं कुम्भः स्वयमुक्तः[3] स्वयम्भुवा ॥ १०१ ॥

nāsā-mūlaṃ mudrayitvā
tad-agre reca-pūrakau ॥
kuryād-utkarṣakaṃ kumbhaḥ
svayam-uktaḥ svayambhuvā ॥ 101 ॥

Tr. Before doing *recaka* and *pūraka*, one should close the nose (at its root) and practise *utkarṣa-kumbhaka* narrated by *svayambhu (śiva)*. 101.

Note. HTK-X.22 referring to some other text (which is not mentioned) describes this technique as follows, - "Holding

1. आरेचपूरौ-HSC. 2. कर्षकं -HSC. 3. स्वयमुक्तं –HSC.

the nose at its root, one should forcefully draw the air in and hold it intensively before one exhales and inhales". 101.

घ्राणार्द्धं[1] मुद्रयित्वाधोभागे यद्रेचपूरकौ ।
कुर्यात्स ब्रह्मणा प्रोक्तः कुम्भको ह्यपकर्षकः ॥ १०२ ॥

ghrāṇārdhaṃ mudrayitvādhobhāge yad-reca-pūrakau ।
kuryāt-sa brahmaṇā proktaḥ kumbhako hyapakarṣakaḥ ॥102॥

Tr. Partially closing the nose and doing *recaka-pūraka* is *apakarṣaka-kumbhaka* stated by *brahmā*. 102.

Note. HTK-X.23 describes this technique as follows:

--Partially closing the nose at its opening, one should inhale and exhale after holding the breath while reciting *praṇava*.

HTK-52:2 provides another technique of *apakarṣa-prāṇāyāma*: Pull up *prāṇa* from the head in a sustained manner through *suṣumnā* and then push it dowanwards. 102.

दीर्घः सूक्ष्मो भवेच्छ्वासः कर्षके कुम्भके कृते ॥ १०३ ॥

dīrghaḥ sūkṣmo bhavec-chvāsaḥ
karṣake kumbhake kṛte ॥ 103 ॥

Tr. With the practice of *karṣaka-kumbhaka (utkarṣa* and *apakarṣaka*), the breath becomes prolonged and subtle. 103.

नोभ्यामारं समाकृष्य कुण्डल्याः पार्श्वयोः[2] क्षिपेत् ।[3]
गच्छता[4] तिष्ठता श्वासधारणं न बलाद्यदा ॥
अनिशं सहजः कुम्भः प्रोक्तः श्रीकृत्तिवाससा ॥ १०४ ॥

nobhyām-āraṃ samākṛṣya kuṇḍalyāḥ pārśvayoḥ kṣipet ।
gacchatā tiṣṭhatā śvāsa-dhāraṇaṃ na balād-yadā ॥
aniśaṃ sahajaḥ kumbhaḥ proktaḥ śrī-kṛttivāsasā ॥ 104 ॥

Tr. Inhaling *prāṇa* through the nose and carrying it along the *kuṇḍalī*, one should hold it comfortably off and on. This is *sahaja-kumbhaka* narrated by *śrī-kṛttivāsa (śiva)*. 104.

1. घोर्द्धं, घोणार्द्धं -J. 2. पार्श्वयो-J. 3. Line not in A. 4. गच्छतो –HSC.

नाडीशुद्धिं तथारोग्यं सुसुखं दीर्घजीवनम्[1] ।
नाद[2]श्रुतिः पापनाशः सहजाभ्यासतो भवेत् ॥ १०५ ॥

nāḍīśuddhiṃ tathārogyaṃ susukhaṃ dīrgha-jīvanam ।
nādaśrutiḥ pāpa-nāśaḥ sahajābhyāsato bhavet ॥ 105 ॥

Tr. With the practice of this *sahaja-kumbhaka,* one gets purification of the *nāḍīs*, health, longevity, hearing of the mystical sounds and removal of all the blemishes. 105.

दक्षवामावर्त्तभेदाच्चक्रशंखौ द्विधोदितौ ॥ १०६ ॥

dakṣa-vāmāvarta-bhedāc-cakra-śaṅkhau dvidhoditau ।106।

Tr. By the distinction of right and left, *cakra* and *śaṅkha kumbhakas* become two-fold. 106.

सूर्येणापूर्य मरुतं कुम्भयेदुदरस्थितम् ।
रेचयेदिन्दुना भूयस्तथा दक्षेण पूरयेत् ॥
कुम्भयेदिडया रिच्या[3]द्दक्षिणावर्त्तचक्रकः ॥ १०७ ॥

sūryeṇāpūrya marutaṃ kumbhayed-udara-sthitam ।
recayed-indunā bhūyas-tathā dakṣeṇa pūrayet ॥
kumbhayed-iḍayā ricyād-dakṣiṇāvartta-cakrakaḥ ॥ 107 ॥

Tr. Taking breath through *sūrya-nāḍī* (right nostril) and after retaining it in the cavity, one should exhale through *indu-nāḍī* (left nostril). Then again one should inhale through the right nostril and exhale through the left nostril after retention. This is *dakṣiṇāvatra-cakra-kumbhaka*. 107.

Note. There does not seem to be any difference in the technique of *dakṣiṇāvartta-cakra-kumbhaka* and *sūrya-bhedana.* The difference lies only in their names. 107.

विलोमोऽयं[4] चक्रकुम्भो[5] वामावर्त्तः शिवोदितः ॥ १०८ ॥

vilomo'yaṃ cakrakumbho vāṃāvartaḥ śivoditaḥ ॥ 108 ॥

Tr. Doing it in the reverse order, it is called *vāmāvarta* (*cakra-kumbhaka*) by *śiva*. 108.

---

1. दीर्घजीविनां –J. 2. नादः -HSC. 3. रेच्य-HSC. 4. विलोपोयं–HSC, विलोमो–J. 5. पञ्चककुम्भो–J.

Note. It is assumed that *vāmāvartta-cakra-kumbhaka* being just opposite to *dakṣiṇāvartta-cakra-kumbhaka*, the technique involves inhalation through the left nostril and exhalation through the right after retention and once again repeating the same technique. This seems to be similar to *candra-bhedana*. 108.

सूर्यचन्द्राविमौ[1] कुम्भौ द्रुहिणेन[2] पुरोदितौ ।
अत्युष्णशीतालावेतौ देशकालप्रयोजितौ[3] ॥ १०९ ॥

sūrya-candrāvimau kumbhau druhiṇena puroditau ।
atyuṣṇa-śītalāvetau deśa-kāla-prayojitau ॥ 109 ॥

Tr. According to *druhiṇa (śiva)*, these are called *sūrya* and *candra kumbhakas* respectively. These being of the nature of heat and cold, they should be practised taking into consideration the region and season. 109.

Note. *jyotsnā* on HP-II.65 gives an elaborate account of the hot and cold effect of the *kumbhakas*. According to *jyotsnā*, in general, all the *kumbhakas* are conducive to all types of people in all seasons and regions. But, *sūrya-bhedana* and *ujjāyī* are prticularly heat generating and therefore are more suitable in cold season. *sītkārī* and *śītalī* are generally suitable in hot seasons. *bhastrā-kumbhaka* is moderate, hence suites in all seasons. Moreover, all the *kumbhakas* have therapeutic values. Even then *sūrya-bhedana* alleviates *vāta* disorders while *ujjāyī* removes phlegmatic conditions. *sītkārī* and *śītalī* are indicated in phlegmatic (*kapha*) conditions. And *bhastrikā-kumbhaka* brings about a balanced condition for all the three *doṣas* (humours). 109.

चक्रकुम्भं द्विधा कुर्यादग्निषोमं तथैकधा ।
शंखकुम्भोऽयमीशेन पूर्ववद् द्विविधः स्मृतः ॥ ११० ॥

cakra-kumbhaṃ dvidhā kuryād-
agniṣomaṃ tathaikadhā ॥
śaṅkha-kumbho'yam-īśena
pūrvavad dvividhaḥ smṛtaḥ ॥ 110 ॥

---

1. चन्द्रसूर्याविमौ-HSC, सूर्याचन्द्राविमौ –HTK. 2. डुहिणेन-J. 3. प्रयाजिकौ-HSC.

Tr. *cakra-kumbhaka* should be practised twice while *agni-ṣoma* one. *śaṅkha-kumbhaka* is also described two-fold as *cakra-kumbhaka* explained before. 110.

Note. *śaṅkha-kumbhaka* has also been stated to be two-fold as *dakṣiṇāvartta* and *vāmāvartta* as indicated by the term `*pūrva-vat*', which means `as before'. 110.

कौष्म्यमी[1]षच्छीतलता कुम्भयोरनयोर्भवेत् ॥ १११ ॥

kauṣmyam-īṣac-chitalatā kumbhayor-anayor-bhavet ॥111॥

Tr. With these two varieties of *kumbhaka*, one experiences warmth and cold. 111.

Note. After the description of *śaṅkha-kumbhaka*, HSC quotes from KP the following additional verse about the technique of *vāma-gati-kumbhaka:-*

"*ubhābhyāṃ pūrayed vāyuṃ kumbhayitvā yathā-vidhi /*
ubhābhyāṃ recayed vāma-gati-kumbhoditaś śivaḥ //

—One should inhale through both the nostrils and after holding the breath systematically, exhale through both the nostrils. This is *vāma-gati-kumbhaka.*"

The same has been described in HTK-X.28 under the name of *vartma-gati-kumbhaka.*

This description is not found in the present text. 111.

उभाभ्यां पूरणं यत्र रेचनं सूर्यवर्त्मना ।
गदाकुम्भः शिवेनोक्तो योगिनो[2] बलकारकः ॥ ११२ ॥

ubhābhyāṃ pūraṇaṃ yatra recanaṃ sūrya-vartmanā ।
gadā-kumbhaḥ śivenokto yogino bala-kārakaḥ ॥ 112 ॥

Tr. Inhalation through both the nostrils and exhalation through the right nostril (*sūrya-nāḍī)* is called *gadā-kumbhaka* by *śiva*, which gives vigour to the *yogīs*. 112.

Note. HTK-X.29 quotes similar technique of *gadā-kumbhaka* from another source which is not mentioned. 112.

---

1. कोष्ण –HSC. 2. योगिनां –HSC.

हं सूर्यो रेफ इत्युक्तः स[1] सोमः[2] च स्मृतो बुधैः ।
सानुस्वारौ बीजमन्त्रौ सिद्धिदौ योगिनाविमौ ॥ ११३ ॥

haṃ sūryo repha ityuktaḥ sa somaḥ ca smṛto budhaiḥ ।
sānusvārau bīja-mantrau siddhidau yogināvimau ॥ 113 ॥

Tr. According to the learned, *ha* represents *sūrya* which is situated below, while *sa* represents *soma (candra)*. With the addition of nasal sound, these become *bīja-mantras* (*haṃ, raṃ* and *saṃ*), which lead the *yogīs* to success. 113.

एकयापूर्य परया[3] रेचनाद्धंसचिन्तनात्[4] ।
यथाशक्त्या निरुध्याथ[5] पूर्य[6] रेचितया पुनः ॥ ११४ ॥

ekayāpūrya parayā recanād-haṃsa-cintanāt ।
yathā-śaktyā nirudhyātha pūrya recitayā punaḥ ॥ 114 ॥

Tr. One should inhale through one nostril and after holding the breath to the capacity, exhale through the other nostril while contemplating on *haṃsa*. Again inhale through the nostril through which one has exhaled. 114.

Note. `*ha*' and `*sa*' are the technical terms in *yoga* symbolically representing sun and moon which suggests the two polarities. The term *haṃsa* represents activity of *prāṇa* and when it is nasalised, *ha* represents exhalatory phase while *sa* represents inhalatory phase. As quoted in the following verse of GhS-V.79 *"hakāreṇa bahir-yāti sakāreṇa viśet punaḥ"*. In the present verse, the exhalatory and inhalatory phases are indicated by alternate nostrils. The term `*haṃsa-cintana*' refers to the conscious observation of the phases of inhalation with *saṃ* and exhalation with *haṃ* through alternate nostrils along with retention. This leads to purification of *nāḍīs*. 113-114.

एवं नाड्योर्विभेदेन चतुःकालेषु[7] विंशतिः ।
कुम्भकान् यदि कुर्वीत नाडीशुध्याख्यकुम्भकः[8] ॥ ११५ ॥

---

1. सः -J. 2. सोमो –J. 3. पूर्वपरया-HSC. 4. रेचकत्वं स चिन्तनात्-HSC. 5. निरुध्यत –HSC. 6. पूर्व –HSC. 7. चतुःकालेति-HSC. 8. शुध्याख्य–A.

evaṃ nāḍyor-vibhedena
catuḥ-kāleṣu viṃśatiḥ ॥
kumbhakān yadi kurvīta
nāḍī-śudhyākhya-kumbhakaḥ ॥ 115 ॥

Tr. When this is parctised with alternate nostrils with twenty *kumbhakas* four times a day, this is known as *(nāḍī-)śuddhi-kumbhaka.* 115.

Note. *nāḍī-śuddhi-kumbhaka* has been described in HTK-X.30 as follows:-

"*haṃseti vindvā manu dvayābhyāṃ*
sve haṃsa-cintanato manasvī ॥
āpūrya mucyed ravi-śītagubhyāṃ
nāḍīviśuddhyākhya kumbhaka eṣaḥ ॥

—While concentrating on *haṃsa*, one should inhale through both the nostrils and after retention should exhale through both the nostrils. This is *nāḍī-śuddhi-kumbhaka.* 115.

See *mārtaṇḍa-kumbhaka* in HTK-X.31. 115.

ग्रीष्ममध्यन्दिनार्द्धाभं नाभौ[1] सवितृमण्डलम् ।
सूर्यनाड्या कृते कुम्भे ध्यात्वा शुध्यन्ति नाडिकाः ॥ ११६ ॥

grīṣma-madhyandinārdhābhaṃ
nābhau savitṛ-maṇḍalam ॥
sūrya-nāḍyā kṛte kumbhe
dhyātvā śuddhyanti nāḍikāḥ ॥ 116 ॥

Tr. When one practises *kumbhaka* after inhaling through the right nostril and concentrating in the navel on the orb of the mid-day sun of the summer, all the *nāḍīs* are purified. 116.

Note. See *mārtaṇḍa-kumbhaka* in HTK-X.31. 116.

शरद्राकानिशीथेन्दुं सहस्रदलमध्यगम् ।
स्रवत् सुधामिडा कुम्भे ध्यात्वा शुध्यन्ति नाडिकाः[2] ॥ ११७ ॥

śaradrākāniśīthenduṃ sahasra-dala-madhyagam ।
sravat sudhām-iḍā kumbhe dhyātvā śudhyanti nāḍikāḥ ।117।

1. ग्रीष्ममध्यं विनाकाभिनामो –HSC. 2. नाडिका-J.

Tr. During the *kumbhaka*, after inhaling through the left nostril, one should visualize oozing of the nectar from the moon of the autumn night, situated in the lotus of the thousand petals (*sahasra-dala*). This leads to purification of the *nāḍīs*. 117.

चन्द्रेण पित्तदोषाणामितरेषां परेण तु ।
नाशः सर्वात्मना भूयात् त्रिभिर्मासैर्न संशयः ॥ ११८ ॥

candreṇa pitta-doṣāṇām-itareṣāṃ pareṇa tu ।
nāśaḥ sarvātmanā bhūyāt tribhir-māsair-na saṃśayaḥ ।118।

Tr. *candra* (inhaling through left nostril) and holding (KP-117) alleviates vitiation of bile (*pitta*), while other (*sūrya-kumbhaka*-KP-116) overcomes other (*kapha* and *vāta*) disorders in three months, in which there is no doubt. 118.

Note. Other techniques of purification of *nāḍīs* have been described in these verses. According to HTK-X.33, all the four techniques described above lead to *nāḍī-śuddhi* which has been specially mentioned. 116-118.

नादश्रुतिः[1] वपुःकार्श्यमारोग्यं वह्निदीपनम् ।
नैर्मल्यमक्ष्णोर्वदनप्रसादो बिन्दुनिर्जयः ॥ ११९ ॥

nāda-śrutiḥ vapuḥ-kārśyam-ārogyaṃ vahni-dīpanam ।
nairmalyam-akṣṇer-vadana-prasādo bindu-nirjayaḥ ।119।

द्वासप्तति[2]सहास्राणां नाडीनां मलशोधनम् ।
यथेष्टं[3] धारणं[4] वायोर्विकाराभाव एव च ॥ १२० ॥

dvāsaptati-sahasrāṇāṃ nāḍīnāṃ mala-śodhanam ।
yatheṣṭaṃ dhāraṇaṃ vāyor-vikārābhāva eva ca ॥ 120 ॥

Tr. This practice results in hearing of mystical sounds, slimness of the body, feeling of wellbeing, increase in gastric fire, clarity of vision, lustrous face, control on *bindu*, purification of all the seventy-two thousand *nāḍīs* and capacity to retain breath willfully and absence of all the disorders of *vāta* humour. 119-120.

---

1. नादश्रुति –J. 2. द्विसप्तति-HSC. 3. ममेष्ट-J. 4. धारणे -J.

Note. Compare HP(L)-IV.15,27 for similar effects. 119-120.

अगर्भेषु सगर्भोऽयमुपयुक्तो निवेषितः ।[1]
फलं संक्षेपतः प्रोक्तं शारीरं तु मया पुरा ॥ १२१ ॥

agarbheṣu sagarbho'yam-upayukto niveṣitaḥ ।
phalaṃ saṃkṣepataḥ proktaṃ śārīraṃ tu mayā purā ॥121॥

Tr. Physical benefits of judicious application (practice) of *sagarbha(-prāṇāyāma)* in lieu of *agarbha* has been narrated by me earlier in short. 121.

Note. Although, in this verse a reference to *agarbha* and *sagarbha* has been made, nowhere in the text these are explained. In other texts of *haṭha-yoga* like GhS, we find that *sagarbha* and *agarbha prāṇāyāma* are clearly explained. The description of *sagarbha* and *agarbha* given in GhS-V.48-52 is as follows: - "Siting in *sukhāsana* posture facing the east or the north, contemplate on *brahmā* associated with *rajas* (active principle), red in color and characterized by the letter `*a*' (of *OM*), let the wise (*yogī*) inhale by the left nostril repeating `*a*' 16 times. After inhalation and before cessation of breath, let him perform *uḍḍiyāna*.

"Then contemplate on *hari* associated with *satva* (illuminating principle) of dark complexion and characterized by the letter `*u*' (of *OM* ), perform *kumbhaka* repeating `*u*' 64 times.

"Then contemplating on *śiva*, associated with *tamas* (delusion) of white color and characterized by the letter `*m*' (of *OM*), exhale, as prescribed, by the right nostril repeating `*m*' 32 times.

"Then inhaling through the right nostril, retain the air by performing *kumbhaka* and expel it through the left nostril, repeating the *bīja-mantra* in the way prescribed."

The technique of *agarbha* remains the same except recitation of *bīja-mantra.*

See also Appendix No-1 in GhS.

---

1. Line not in A.

Traditionally we find two types of *kumbhakas*— namely *agarbha* and *sagarbha*. *agarbha* is without *mantra* while *sagarbha* is with *mantra*. *patañjali's prāṇāyāma* is *agarbha*, but requires counting of *mātrās*. In *smārta* way of *sagarbha prāṇāyāma*, one mentally recites a long *mantra* such as *gāyatrī* along with *praṇava*, *vyāhṛti* and *śiras*.

GhS-V.47 describes twofold *sahita-kumbhaka* and calls them *sagarbha* and *nigarbha*. *kumbhaka* performed, while mentally repeating a *bīja-mantra* is *sagarbha* and that without such repetition is *nigarbha*. It also suggests contemplation on `*a*', `*u*' and `*m*' along with meditation on *brahmā*, *hari* and *śiva*. (Also see GhS-V.48-57).

YSC-II.51 describes *sagarbha-prāṇāyāma* as three-fold and calls them *sadhūmaka*, *sajvāla* and *praśānta*. While explaining these terms it says that *sadhūmaka prāṇāyāma* involves recitation of a *mantra* and concentration on its parts for a period of one or three *mātrās*. In *sajvāla prāṇāyāma* the technique involves recitation of a *mantra* and concentration on its parts and their meaning and the deity in its totality. The *praśānta* type of *prāṇāyāma* is without recitation of *mantra* and its parts and without the concentration of any form of the deity devoid of any disposition but contemplation on the inner space in abstract form.

In DB also *prāṇāyāma* is described to be of six types – *sadhūmaka*, *vidhūmaka*, *sagarbha*, *agarbha*, *salakṣya* and *alakṣya*. 121.

तत्वादौ पूरयेद्वायुं तत्तत्वान्ते विरेचयेत् ।
तत्वकुम्भः स गदितः पञ्चधा तत्वभेदतः ॥ १२२ ॥

tatvādau pūrayed-vāyuṃ tat-tatvānte virecayet ।
tatva-kumbhaḥ sa gaditaḥ pañcadhā tatva-bhedataḥ ॥ 122 ॥

Tr. One should inhale before the rise of a particular *tatva* (element) and exhale at the end of that *tatva*. This is called *tatva-kumbhaka* which is five-fold according to the five *tatvas*. 122.

Note. The term *tatva* refers to the five elements called earth, water, fire, air and ether. Full discussion about the *tatvas*, their rise, duration, their properties and application have been elaborately discussed in the traditional text called *śiva-svarodaya.* This information is briefly presented in the table in **Appendix-iii**.

The period of prevalence of *tatvas* differ according to different texts. For example, YSC-I.39 describes the duration of the *tatvas* as double that of *śiva-svarodaya.* 122.

तत्तत्त्वगुणं योगी शीतोष्णकठिनादिकम् ।
लभते तत्वकुम्भेन कुण्डलीबोधनाद्यपि ॥ १२३ ॥

tat-tat-tatva-guṇaṃ yogī śītoṣṇa-kaṭhinādikam ।
labhate tatva-kumbhena kuṇḍalī-bodhanādyapi ॥ 123 ॥

Tr. Through the practice of *tatva-kumbhaka, kuṇḍalinī* is aroused and a *yogī* is able to attain the qualities of a particular *tatva* like cold, heat, hardness etc. 123.

तत्तत्वोदये चापूर्य पञ्चतत्वेषु कुम्भयेत् ।
तत्तत्वोदयने तत्वजयः श्वसनरेचनात् ॥ १२४ ॥

tat-tatvodaye cāpūrya pañca-tatveṣu kumbhayet ।
tat-tatvodayane tatva-jayaḥ śvasana-recanāt ॥ 124 ॥

Tr. On the rise of a particular *tatva*, one should inhale, retain and exhale. This is practised during (the rise of) all the five *tatvas* (elements). This leads to control over the *tatvas.* 124.

तत्तत्त्वजयं कुर्याच्छरीरं दिव्यमद्भूतम्
कुम्भकस्तत्वजयनो मोक्षमार्ग प्रदर्शयेत् ॥ १२५ ॥

tat-tat-tatva-jayaṃ kuryāc-charīraṃ divyam-adbhūtam ।
kumbhakas-tatva-jayano mokṣa-mārgaṃ pradarśayet ।125।

Tr. With the control of the elements, one attains divine body. *kumbhaka* practised during the control of the elements leads to *mokṣa* (liberation). 125.

दिनेशवर्त्मनाकृष्य बाह्यवायुं सशब्दकम् ।
यावद् हृत्कण्ठयोगः स्यादानखाग्रशिखाग्रकम् ॥ १२६ ॥

dineśa-vartmanākṛṣya
bāhya-vāyuṃ saśabdakam ॥
yāvad hṛt-kaṇṭha-yogaḥ syād-
ānakhāgra-śikhāgrakam ॥ 126 ॥

पूरयित्वा यथेष्टं तं कुम्भितं चेडया त्यजेत् ।
सूर्यभेदाख्यकुम्भोऽयं पुनः पुनरिमं चरेत् ॥ १२७ ॥

pūrayitvā yatheṣṭaṃ taṃ
kumbhitaṃ ceḍayā tyajet ॥
sūrya-bhedākhya-kumbho'yaṃ
punaḥ punar-imaṃ caret ॥ 127 ॥

Tr. One should inhale the external air through the right nostril with sound, filling the throat to maximum capacity and exhale through *iḍā* (left nostril), after holding the breath. This is *sūryabhedana-kumbhaka* which should be practised again and again. 126-127.

Note. Similar technique is described in the well-known text of HP(L)-IV.37-39, but there is no mention of inhalation with sound, whereas in this text there is a specific mention of sound during inhalation. 126-127.

अनेन विधिना चन्द्रनाड्योक्तश्चन्द्र[1]भेदतः ॥ १२८ ॥[2]
anena vidhinā candra-nāḍyoktaś-candra-bhedataḥ ॥ 128 ॥

Tr. Similarly, when one practises starting inhalation through *candra-nāḍī* (left nostril), it is called *candra-bhedana.* 128.

उदरे वातदोषघ्नं कृमिहृत्कण्ठदोषनुत् ।
कपालशोधनं सूर्यभेदनं स्यान्न संशयः ॥
औष्ण्यशैत्यकारावेतौ पार्वतीपतिनेरितौ[2] ॥ १२९ ॥[3]
udare vāta-doṣaghnaṃ kṛmi-hṛt-kaṇṭha-doṣanut ।
kapāla-śodhanaṃ sūrya-bhedanaṃ syānna saṃśayaḥ ॥
auṣṇya-śaitya-karāvetau pārvatī-patineritau ॥ 129 ॥
तत्र पुष्टिकरश्चन्द्रभेदाह्वः स्यान्न संशयः ॥ १३० ॥[3]
tatra puṣṭikaraś-candra-bhedāhvaḥ syān-na saṃśayaḥ ।130।

---

1. श्चण्ड –J. 2. पतिनेरितै-J. 3. Verse not in A.

Tr. The practice of *sūrya-bhedana* undoubtedly removes disorders of *vāta* humour in the abdomen, disorders of throat, heart and removes worms and purifies the forehead. Accordiung to *śiva*, these two produce heat and cold respectively. The practice of *candra-bhedana* undoubtedly brings nourishment. 129-130.

मुखं नियम्य नाडीभ्यामाकृष्यासुं नियोजयेत् ।
कुण्डलीपार्श्वयोः पश्चात् कुम्भयेदुदरस्थितम् ॥ १३१ ॥
mukhaṃ niyamya nāḍībhyām-ākṛṣyāsuṃ niyojayet ।
kuṇḍalī-pārśvayoḥ paścāt kumbhayed-udara-sthitam ।131।
रेचयेदिडया[1] वायुं गच्छन्तिष्ठन्यदा चरेत् ।
उज्जायीकुम्भकः प्रोक्तः शिवेनाखिलवेदिना ॥ १३२ ॥
recayed-iḍayā vāyuṃ gacchan-tiṣṭhan-yadā caret ।
ujjāyī-kumbhakaḥ proktaḥ śivenākhilavedinā ॥ 132 ॥

Tr. Closing the mouth, one should inhale air through both the nostrils while holding it along the *kuṇḍalī* and exhale through the left nostril. This is *ujjāyī-kumbhaka* stated by *śiva*, which should be practised all the time. 131-132.

Note. Similar technique is described in HP(L)-IV.40-42 but the inhalation through both the nostrils is performed with frictional sound, which is not mentioned here in this text. 131-132.

गदं[2] बलासं च जलोदरं च
नाड्युत्थदोषं कफजं च कण्ठे ॥
धातुस्थितं दोषगणं निहन्ति
कुर्याच्च दीप्तिं निजदेहवह्नेः ॥ १३३ ॥
gadaṃ balāsaṃ ca jalodaraṃ ca
nāḍyuttha-doṣaṃ kaphajaṃ ca kaṇṭhe ॥
dhātu-sthitaṃ doṣa-gaṇaṃ nihanti
kuryāc-ca dīptiṃ nija-deha-vahneḥ ॥ 133 ॥

1. रेचयेद्रया –J. 2. गरं –A.

Tr. This practice removes disorders of phlegm, dropsy, morbidity of the *nāḍīs* and vitiation of the humours in the *dhātus* (bodily constituents), phlegmatic disorders of the throat and increases bodily fire and luster. 133.

बलादाकर्षयेद्वायुं यावद् घ्राणसुमुद्रणम् ।
कुम्भयेच्च तथा वायुं कुम्भराजोऽयमीरितः ॥ १३४ ॥
balād-ākarṣayed-vāyuṃ yāvad ghrāṇa-sumudraṇam ।
kumbhayec-ca tathā vāyuṃ kumbharājo'yam-īritaḥ ॥134॥

Tr. One should forcefully inhale air and hold the breath by closing the nose properly. This is called *kumbha-rāja.* 134.

कुर्याद्वायुजयं वह्निवृद्धिमेषो हि कुम्भकः ॥ १३५ ॥
kuryād-vāyu-jayaṃ vahni-
vṛddhim-eṣo hi kumbhakaḥ ॥ 135 ॥

Tr. This *kumbhaka* brings control over *vāyu* and increases heat. 135.

क्रियन्तेऽथ समासेन काकचञ्चुभिदः स्फुटाः ।
सीत्कारी प्रथमोऽन्ये तु शीतलीत्यभिधाः स्मृताः ॥ १३६ ॥
kriyante'tha samāsena kākacañcu-bhidaḥ sphuṭāḥ ।
sītkārī prathamo'nye tu śītalītyabhidhāḥ smṛtāḥ ॥ 136 ॥

Tr. Now we describe in nut shell and clearly the techniques called *kāka-cañcu* which are named *sītkārī* by some and *śītalī* by others. 136.

रसनामुन्मुखीकृत्य सीत्कारं कुर्वता मरुत्[1] ।
पीयन्ते कुम्भके यस्मिन् नासिकाभ्यां विरेचनम् ॥ १३७ ॥
rasanām-unmukhīkṛtya sītkāraṃ kurvatā marut ।
pīyante kumbhake yasmin nāsikābhyāṃ virecanam ॥137॥
रसनां प्राणसंयुक्तां पीड्यमानां विचिन्तयेत् ।
सीत्कारीकुम्भकः प्रोक्तः सर्वसिद्धिकरः सताम् ॥ १३८ ॥

1. मकत् –J.

rasanāṃ prāṇa-saṃyuktāṃ pīḍyamānāṃ vicintayet ।
sītkārī-kumbhakaḥ proktaḥ sarva-siddhikaraḥ satām ॥138॥

Tr. Turning the tongue upwards and producing the sound `*sīt*', inhale the air. After holding the breath, exhale through both the nostrils, while making frictional sound. Concentrate on the tongue pressed and the sound along with *prāṇa*. This is called *sītkārī-kumbhaka*, which contributes to all the accomplishements. 137-138.

Note. In these varieties of *kākacañcu* and *sītkārī* air is inhaled through mouth. In all the *prāṇāyāma* techniques air is invariably exhaled and inhaled through the nostrils. *brahmānanda* in *jyotsnā* (HP-II.53) cautions against inhalation through mouth. 136-138.

सीत्कारीकुम्भकाभ्यासात् स्मरजित्वररूपधृक् ।
क्षुन्निद्रालस्यरोगसर्वोपद्रववर्जितः ॥ १३९ ॥
sītkārī-kumbhakābhyāsāt smara-jitvara-rūpa-dhṛk ।
kṣun-nidrālasya-roga-sarvopadrava-varjitaḥ ॥ 139 ॥
योगीन्द्रो योगिनीचक्रसेव्यः सृष्ट्यादिकृत् भवेत् ॥ १४० ॥
yogīndro yoginī-cakra-sevyaḥ sṛṣṭyādi-kṛt bhavet ॥ 140 ॥

Tr. With the practice of *sītkārī-kumbhaka*, one controls the cupid (god of love) and becomes handsome. It helps in controlling hunger, sleep, laziness, diseases and one becomes free from all the problems of health. The *yogī* enjoys the multitude of powers like creation etc. 139-140.

Note. Often the term *yoginī-cakra* may be translated as a group of female partners of the aspirants in *tāntrika* tradition. In this context the meaning conveyed is the group of deities presiding over the *cakras* and their manifestation from *mūlādhāra* to *sahasrāra*. 139-140.

नलिकासदृशीं काकुं विधायापूरयेत्तया ।
श्वसनं[1] कुम्भयेन्नोभ्यां रेचयेत् काकचञ्चुकः ॥ १४१ ॥

---

1. शसनं –J.

nalikāsadṛśīṃ kākuṃ
vidhāyāpūrayet-tayā ॥
śvasanaṃ kumbhayen-nobhyāṃ
recayet kāka-cañcukaḥ ॥ 141 ॥

क्षुत्तृट्पित्तज्वरप्लीहविषाणां नाशनो भवेत् ॥ १४२ ॥
kṣut-tṛṭ-pitta-jvara-plīha-viṣāṇāṃ nāśano bhavet ॥ 142 ॥

Tr. Forming the tongue like a tube, take the air in through it. After holding the breath, exhale through the nose. This is *kāka-cañcu*. It removes hunger, thirst, bilious tendency, fever and inflammation of the spleen and toxicity. 141-142.

काकचञ्चुवदास्येनापूर्य वायुं निरोधयेत् ।
ऊर्ध्वजिह्वां[1] समानीय पिबेद्धारामृतं सुधीः[2] ॥
रेचयेद् घ्राणरन्ध्राभ्यां[3] शीतलीकाकचञ्चुकः ॥ १४३ ॥
kākacañcu-vad-āsyaenāpūrya vāyuṃ nirodhayet ।
ūrdhvajihvāṃ samānīya pibed-dhārāmṛtaṃ sudhīḥ ॥
recayed ghrāṇa-randhrābhyāṃ śītalī-kākacañcukaḥ ।143।

Tr. Forming the mouth like the beak of a crow, one should take the air in and hold it. Then raising the tongue, one should taste the flow of nectar and exhale through both the nostrils. This is *śītalī-kāka-cañcuka*. 143.

Note. *śītalī-prāṇāyāma* is also named as *kāka-cañcuka* here. 143.

प्राणापानविधानज्ञो मुक्तिभागस्य साधनात् ।
नित्याभ्यासवतो याति श्रमदाहज्वरामयाः ॥
मासाभ्यासान्मृत्युजयो निरन्तरकृते भवेत् ॥ १४४ ॥
prāṇāpāna-vidhānajño muktibhāg-asya sādhanāt ।
nityābhyāsavato yāti śrama-dāha-jvarāmayāḥ ॥
māsābhyāsān-mṛtyu-jayo nirantara-kṛte bhavet ॥ 144 ॥

---

1. ऊर्ध्वां जिह्वां-J. 2. सुखी-HTK. 3. घ्राणसन्धाभ्यां –HTK.

Tr. An adept of *prāṇa* and *apāna* practises this consistently for a month gets rid of heat due to exertion, fever and other sickness and overcomes premature death. 144.

मणिकर्णिबिलं गाढं[1] पीड्य लम्बिकया ततः ।
कुण्डलीं चिन्तयन्[2] काकचञ्च्वा यदि समीरणम् ॥
पिबेत् षण्मासयोगेन कविर्भवति निश्चितम् ॥१४५॥
maṇikarṇi-bilaṃ gāḍhaṃ pīḍya lambikayā tataḥ ।
kuṇḍalīṃ cintayan kāka-cañcvā yadi samīraṇam ॥
pibet ṣaṇmāsa-yogena kavir-bhavati niścitam ॥ 145 ॥

Tr. Turning the tip of the tongue up and pressing it to the throat, one should take the air through the mouth forming it like the beak of a crow and contemplate on *kuṇḍalī*. Practising this for six months, one undoubtedly becomes a *kavi* (poet). 145.

ध्यात्वा कुण्डलिनीवक्त्रगामिनं[3] मारुतं यदा ।
काकचञ्चुं प्रकुरुते क्षयरोगात् प्रमुच्यते ॥ १४६ ॥
dhyātvā kuṇḍalinī-vaktra-gāminaṃ mārutaṃ yadā ।
kāka-cañcuṃ prakurute kṣaya-rogāt pramucyate ॥ 146 ॥
दूरश्रुतिर्दूरदृष्टिरन्तर्द्धानादिकं फलम् ।
अहर्निशं सदाभ्यासाज्जायते नात्र संशयः ॥ १४७ ॥
dūra-śrutir-dūra-dṛṣṭir-antardhānādikaṃ phalam ।
ahar-niśaṃ sadābhyāsāj-jāyate nātra saṃśayaḥ ॥ 147 ॥

Tr. Forming the tongue into the beak of a crow one should take the air in and contemplate on *prāṇa* entering into the mouth of *kuṇḍalī*. With this, one becomes free from the disease of consumption. With daily and continuous practice, one undoubtedly attains clairaudience, foresightedness and ability to disappear. 146-147.

---

1. काकुजिह्वां-J. 2. चिन्तयेत् –HTK. 3. चक्रगामिनं –HSC.

द्विजैर्द्विजान् पीड्य वायुं काकचञ्च्वा[1] पिबेच्छनैः ।
ऊर्ध्वजिह्वः कुम्भकारो रेचयेद् घ्राणवर्त्मना ॥
काकचञ्चुः कुम्भ उक्तः केनायं काकुदश्रवाः[2] ॥ १४८ ॥

dvijair-dvijān pīḍya vāyuṃ kākacañcvā pibec-chanaiḥ ।
ūrdhva-jihvaḥ kumbhakāro recayed ghrāṇa-vartmanā ॥
kākacañcuḥ kumbha uktaḥ kenāyaṃ kākudaśravāḥ ॥148॥

Tr. By pressing the teeth together, one should take the air in slowly through the mouth and holding the breath with upturned tongue, exhale through the passage of nose. According to *kākudaśravā* this is *kāka-cañcu-kumbhaka.* 148.

आवत्सरार्द्धमभ्यासं प्रत्यहं यः समाचरेत् ।
सर्वरोगविनिर्मुक्तो वत्सरान् मृत्युजिद् भवेत् ॥ १४९ ॥

āvatsarārdham-abhyāsaṃ pratyahaṃ yaḥ samācaret ।
sarva-roga-vinirmukto vatsarān mṛtyu-jid bhavet ॥ 149 ॥

Tr. By daily practice of this *kumbhaka* for half a year, one completely gets rid of the diseases and after a year (of practice) one controls (premature) death. 149.

त्रिवर्षे[3] शिवतां याति भूतेन्द्रियजयान्वितः ।
अणिमादिगुणैर्युक्तो जरया रहितो भवेत् ॥ १५० ॥

tri-varṣe śivatāṃ yāti bhūtendriya-jayānvitaḥ ।
āṇimādi-guṇair-yukto jarayā rahito bhavet ॥ 150 ॥

खेचर्यंगमिदं[4] प्राह कृपालुः परमेश्वरः ॥ १५१ ॥

khecaryaṅgamidaṃ prāha kṛpāluḥ parameśvaraḥ ॥ 151 ॥

Tr. Having controlled all the senses and accomplishing *siddhis* like *aṇimā* etc., one overcomes signs of old age and attains *śiva*-hood after three years. It is the means leading to *khecarī,* (an undisturbed state of consciousness), as narrated by *parameśvara* the merciful. 150-151.

---

1. काकचञ्चा-HSC. 2. केनाथ काकुदश्रवा –HSC. 3. त्रिवर्षैः -HTK. 4. खेचर्यं गतिदं –HTK.

Note. *khecarī* here refers to undisturbed state of consciousness. 150-151.

श्रद्धालुसुकुम्भकाश्च क्षुत्तृडादिविनाशिनः ।
सर्वसौभाग्यधातारो विज्ञेयाः गुरुवाक्यतः ॥ १५२ ॥[1]

śraddhālu-sukumbhakāś-ca kṣut-tṛḍādi-vināśinaḥ ।
sarva-saubhāgya-dhātāro vijñeyāḥ guru-vākyataḥ ॥ 152 ॥

Tr. *kumbhakas* practised with devotion remove hunger and thirst and contribute to all fortunes, which should be learnt from the *guru*. 152.

मात्राः षोडशपूरे स्युश्चतुःषष्ट्यस्तु कुम्भके[2] ।
द्वात्रिंशद्रेचके प्रोक्ताः मात्राकुम्भः समीरितः ॥ १५३ ॥

mātrāḥ ṣoḍaśa-pūre syuś-catuḥ-ṣaṣṭyas-tu kumbhake ।
dvātriṃśad-recake proktāḥ mātrākumbhaḥ samīritaḥ ॥153॥

Tr. Inhaling air for sixteen *mātrās* (time units) and holding it for sixty-four *mātrās* and exhaling for thirty-two *mātrās* is known as *mātrā-kumbhaka*. 153.

Note. The special feature of *mātrā-kumbhaka* seems to be the ratio of 16: 64: 32 units of time, for *pūraka, kumbhaka* and *recaka* respectively. 153.

मात्राकुम्भो[3] हृदि कृतः[4] शोषकः सम्प्रकीर्त्तितः ।
दाहनो नाभिसंस्थानो मात्राकुम्भः प्रकीर्त्तितः ॥ १५४ ॥

mātrā-kumbho hṛdi kṛtaḥ śoṣakaḥ samprakīrtitaḥ ।
dāhano nābhi-saṃsthāno mātrākumbhaḥ prakīrtitaḥ ॥154॥

Tr. If *mātrā-kumbhaka* is practised in the chest region, it causes absorption and parctised in the navel region, it generates heat. 154.

स्वाधिष्ठानानुगश्चायं[5] प्लावनो[6]ऽमृतसेचनः ।
मूलाधारे कृतश्चायं[7] कठिनीकरणो[8] मतः ॥ १५५ ॥

---

1. Verse not in A. 2. चतुःषष्ट्या सुकुम्भके –HSC. 3. मात्राकुम्भे –HSC. 4. मात्राकुम्भायाम एष –HTK. 5. सोयं –HTK. 6. प्लवनो –HTK. 7. कृतश्चामं –J. 8. कठिनाकरणे –HTK.

svādhiṣṭhānanugaś-cāyaṃ plāvano'mṛta-secanaḥ ।
mūlādhāre kṛtaś-cāyaṃ kaṭhinī-karaṇo mataḥ ॥ 155 ॥

Tr. When it is practised in *svādhiṣṭhāna*, it increases the flow of nectar, when practised in *mūlādhāra*, one attains stability. 155.

पुनः कण्ठानुगो पञ्च व्यूहनः[1] स्यात् स कुम्भकः ।
ब्रह्मस्थाननियोगेन[2] मुक्तिदः परिकीर्त्तितः[3] ॥ १५६ ॥
punaḥ kaṇṭhānugo pañca vyūhanaḥ syāt sa kumbhakaḥ ।
brahma-sthāna-niyogena muktidaḥ parikīrtitaḥ ॥ 156 ॥

Tr. When parctised in the region of throat, this *kumbhaka* balances the five *bhūtas* and practised in the *brahmasthāna* (region of *brahmarandhra*), it leads to emancipation. 156.

रुध्वा घोणायुगं कुर्याद्युगपद्यदि षट्क्रमात् ।
भूतशुद्धिरिति प्रोक्त आदिनाथेन शम्भुना ॥ १५७ ॥
ruddhvā ghoṇā-yugaṃ kuryād-yugapad-yadi ṣaṭ-kramāt ।
bhūta-śuddhir-iti prokta ādināthena śambhunā ॥ 157 ॥

Tr. According to *ādinātha (śambhu)*, if this *kumbhaka* is practised simultaneously in the six regions (stated above) in progression, it leads to purification of the *bhūtas*. 157.

मात्रा नवविधा प्रोक्ता योगिभिस्तत्वदर्शिभिः ।
निमेषोन्मेषणं[4] मात्राकालो लघ्वक्षरान्वितः[5] ॥ १५८ ॥
mātrā nava-vidhā proktā yogibhis-tatva-darśibhiḥ ।
nimeṣonmeṣaṇaṃ mātrākālo laghvakṣarānvitaḥ ॥ 158 ॥
मिता द्वादशह्रस्वानां शीघ्रमुच्चारकालतः ।
प्रदक्षिणीकृत्य जानुं न द्रुतं[6] न विलम्बितम्[7] ॥ १५९ ॥

---

1. कण्ठानुगो पंचेषूहनः -HTK. 2. ब्रह्मस्थानेन योगेन –HSC. ब्रह्मस्थाननियोगेन –HTK. 3. प्रकीर्त्तितः -J. 4. निमेषोन्मेषणे –HSC. 5. लघ्वक्षरोन्मितः -J. 6. द्रूतं –HTK. 7. जानुनातिद्रुतविलम्बितं –HTK. जानुं न द्रूतं विलम्बितं –HTK.

mitā dvādaśa-hrasvānāṃ śīghram-uccāra-kālataḥ ।
pradakṣiṇī-kṛtya jānuṃ na drutaṃ na vilambitam ॥ 159 ॥

अंगुलीत्रिकतो मात्रा छोटिकाकरणाद् भवेत् ।
गोदोहवत्सपानेषु क्षेपघण्टारवोन्मिता[1] ॥ १६० ॥

aṅgulī-trikato mātrā choṭikā-karaṇād bhavet ।
godoha-vatsa-pāneṣu kṣepaghaṇṭā-ravonmitā ॥ 160 ॥

Tr. The learned *yogīs* state the measure of time, called *mātrā,* to be nine-fold. The measure of *mātrā* is—(i) time taken for twinkling of the eyes, (ii) pronouncing a short vowel, (iii) time taken for quick pronunciation of 12 short vowels, (iv) going round the knee-joint with hand neither too slow nor too fast, (v) snapping together three fingers, (vi) ringing of the bell when feeding the calf at the time of milking a cow. 158-160.

Note. According to the tradition of *tantra*, *choṭikā* is a syllable standing for *phaṭ*. 158-160.

चतुरो ह्यतिमात्रा[2] स्युस्ताश्च[3] सेव्याः शनैः शनैः ।
देशकालानुसारेण प्राहुर्योगीश्वराः पुराः ॥ १६१ ॥

caturo hyatimātrā syus-tāś-ca sevyāḥ śanaiḥ śanaiḥ ।
deśa-kālānusāreṇa prāhur-yogīśvarāḥ purāḥ ॥ 161 ॥

Tr. There are four other varieties narrated by the ancient *yogīs*, called *atimātrās* which are to be used gradually according to the region and season. 161.

पूरकुम्भकरेचेषु निसर्गजनितेषु यः[4] ।
कालः स मात्रासंज्ञः स्यात् स्वस्वमानक्रमादिमाः ॥ १६२ ॥

pūra-kumbhaka-receṣu nisarga-janiteṣu yaḥ ।
kālaḥ sa mātrā-saṃjñaḥ syāt sva-sva-māna-kramād-imāḥ ।162।

Tr. The duration of the time taken for *pūraka*, *kumbhaka* and *recaka* by the individual according to his natural capacity is also called *mātrā*. 162.

---

1. मिताः -J, HSC. 2. ह्यतिमात्राः -HTK. 3. तासु –HSC. 4. निसर्गजनिषेमः -A,J.

अ उ मा इति ताश्चैव महामात्राः पुरोदिताः ॥ १६३ ॥

a-u-mā iti tāś-caiva mahā-mātrāḥ puroditāḥ ॥ 163 ॥

Tr. *a*, *u* and *mā* are regarded as *mahāmātrā* from ancient times. 163.

Note. In ancient times, in the absence of watches *yogis* devised particular time units and called them *mātrās*. Different schools had different time values assigned to the *mātrās*. An examination of the *yogic* literature reveals the fact that there was no uniformity in understanding the time value of *mātrās*. According to SPu, the time taken for one respiration is the time value of a *mātrā*. *bhāskarācārya*, the great Indian astronomer, has the following table of time units-

6 respirations	= 1 *pala*
60 *palas*	= 1 *ghaṭikā*
60 *ghaṭikās*	= 24 hours

Working with this table, we find that each respiration takes four seconds. Thus, here we get definite time value for *mātrā*.

In MPu :-

1 *mātrā* = time taken for twinkling of the eye or pronouncing a short vowel (2 seconds)

15 twinklings	= 1 *kāṣṭhā* (3.2 seconds)
30 *kāṣṭhās*	= 1 *kalā* (96 seconds)
30 *kalās*	= 1 *muhūrta* (48 minutes)
30 *muhūrtas*	= 1 day and night (24 hours)

BYS and SPu define *mātrā* in the form of an equation as follows:-

Once snapping the thumb and the fore finger	Once going round = the knee joint with the hand	Three claps = (SPu)
Thrice snapping the thumb and the fore finger	Thrice going = round the knee-joint with hand	Three claps = (BYS-VIII.12-13)

Thus we find the inconsistencies of time units (*mātrās*) followed by different schools.

Here in this text also nine different types of *mātrās* have been mentioned, but on counting them, they do not fulfill the number of nine.

Even the *mātrās* that are described, are not consistent. Thus we find no uniformity regarding the measure of *mātrā*. 158-163.

भस्त्रेव लोहकारस्य रेचपूरौ श्रमावधि ।
वेगेन स्तनयोरूर्ध्वं ततः पूरोऽर्कवर्त्मना ॥ १६४ ॥

bhastreva loha-kārasya reca-pūrau śramāvadhi ।
vegena stanayor-ūrdhvaṃ tataḥ pūro'rka-vartmanā ॥164॥

जालन्धरं दृढं बध्वा कुम्भितं चन्द्रवर्त्मना ।
रेचयेद् भस्त्रिकाकुम्भः शरीराग्निविवर्द्धनः ॥ १६५ ॥

jālandharaṃ dṛḍhaṃ baddhvā
kumbhitaṃ candra-vartmanā ॥
recayed bhastrikā-kumbhaḥ
śarīrāgni-vivardhanaḥ ॥ 165 ॥

वातपित्तकफहृत्कजवातं हन्ति गीर्मुखकपाटममोघः ।
शक्तिबोधजनकस्त्रितयात्मग्रन्थिनिपुणः सुखदोऽयम् ॥१६६॥

vāta-pitta-kapha-hṛt-kaja-vātaṃ
hanti gīr-mukha-kapāṭam-amoghaḥ ।
śaktibodha-janakas-tritayātma-
granthi-nipuṇaḥ sukhado'yam ॥ 166 ॥

Tr. One should exhale and inhale like the bellows of a blacksmith until fatigue sets in. Then he should rapidly inhale through the right nostril and exhale through the left nostril, after holding the breath performing *jālandhara-bandha*. It is *bhastrikā-kumbhaka*.

This increases bodily heat and removes disorders of the three humours called *vāta, pitta* and *kapha*. One becomes proficient in speech and learning and gets *kuṇḍalinī* aroused which pierces the three knots and bestows happiness. 164-166.

Note. Similar technique has been described in HP(L)-IV.50-56. 164-165.

नासाग्रमुद्रणं कृत्वा यदन्ता रेचपूरकौ ।
पूर्ववत् कुम्भकं कुर्यादन्तर्भस्त्रेयमीरिता ॥ १६७ ॥

nāsāgra-mudraṇaṃ kṛtvā yadantā reca-pūrakau ।
pūrvavat kumbhakaṃ kuryād-antar-bhastreyam-īritā ॥167॥

Tr. By closing one nostril, practise exhalation and inhalation to the capacity and hold the breath as stated earlier (before exhalation). This is called *antar-bhastrā*. 167.

Note. The technique described here is not clear. However, *brahmānanda* in his *jyotsnā* on HP-II.59-64 while commenting on *bhastrikā*, gives different traditions, out of which one tradition fits with the technique given here. The detailed technique of this *antar-bhastrā* can be described as follows: -

" Closing the left nostril by little and ring fingers one should exhale and inhale with the right nostril rapidly like the bellows. When the fatigue sets in, inhale through the same (right) nostril and closing both the nostrils, hold the breath to the capacity and then exhale through the left nostril. This technique may be reversed substituting or changing the nostrils." 167.

सकृद् रेचपूराभ्यां कुम्भोऽयं चान्तरंगकः ॥ १६८ ॥
sakṛd reca-pūrābhyāṃ kumbho'yaṃ cantaraṅgakaḥ ॥168॥

Tr. Retaining the breath after sudden exhalation and inhalation is *antaraṅga-kumbhaka*. 168.

Note. *brahmānanda* also gives another tradition of *bhastrikā* which fits in the technique described under *antaraṅga bhastrikā*. This technique can be described as follows-

"Closing the left nostril with the little and the ring fingers, quickly inhale through the right nostril and suddenly closing the right nostril with the thumb, quickly exhale through the left nostril. Repeating this for several times, inhale through the right nostril and holding the breath with *jālandhara-bandha*, exhale through the left nostril. This process may be reversed by changing the nostrils". (*brahmānanda's* commentary *jyotsnā* on HP-II.59-64). 168.

अलिशब्दयुतं वेगात् पूरयेत् कुम्भयेत्ततः ।
सालिशब्दाच्छनै रेकात् भ्रामरीकुम्भको मुनेः ॥
आनन्दलीलां कुरुते भ्रामरीकुम्भको मुनेः ॥ १६९ ॥

ali-śabda-yutaṃ vegāt pūrayet kumbhayet-tataḥ ।
sāli-śabdāc-chanai rekāt bhrāmarī-kumbhako muneḥ ॥
ānanda-līlāṃ kurute bhrāmarī-kumbhako muneḥ ॥ 169 ॥

Tr. Inhale rapidly producing the sound of a black bee and exhale slowly with the sound of a black bee after retaining the breath. This is called *bhrāmarī-kumbhaka* which produces ecstasy. 169.

आपूर्य कुम्भितं प्राणं बध्वा जालन्धरं शनैः ॥
रेचयेन्मूर्च्छनाकुम्भो मनोमूर्च्छा सुखप्रदा[1] ॥ १७० ॥

āpūrya kumbhitaṃ prāṇaṃ
baddhvā jālandharaṃ śanaiḥ ॥
recayen-mūrcchanā-kumbho
mano-mūrcchā sukha-pradā ॥ 170 ॥

Tr. The inhaled air is retained with *jālandhara-bandha* and exhaled slowly while maintaining *jālandhara-bandha*. It is called *mūrcchanā-kumbhaka* which brings enjoyable tranquility of the mind. 170.

Note. For a similar technique of *mūrchanā-kumbhaka* see HP(L)-IV.69. 170.

यथेष्टं पूरयेद्वायुं बद्धे जालन्धरे दृढे ।
हृदि धृत्वा जले सुप्त्वा प्लाविनीकुम्भको भवेत् ॥ १७१ ॥

yatheṣṭaṃ pūrayed-vāyuṃ baddhe jālandhare dṛḍhe ।
hṛdi dhṛtvā jale suptvā plāvinī-kumbhako bhavet ॥ 171 ॥

फलके प्लवनानन्दः कुम्भकश्च निगद्यते ॥ १७२ ॥

phalake plavanānandaḥ kumbhakaś-ca nigadyate ॥ 172 ॥

Tr. After taking the air in and adopting *jālandhara-bandha*, when one lies in the water, it becomes *plāvinī-kumbhaka*. This *kumbhaka* gives the pleasure as if one floats on a wooden plank. 171-172.

Note. The technique of *plāvinī-kumbhaka* described in HP-II.70 requires the stomach to be filled with air but there is no mention of *jālandhara-bandha*. 171-172.

---

1. सुखप्रदः -J.

शृंखलाजीवचालमेरुश्चेति[1] रहस्यकम् ।
विहायान्येषु कुम्भेषु किमर्थमनुधावनम्[2] ॥ १७३ ॥
śṛṅkhalā-jīva-cāla-meruś-ceti rahasyakam ।
vihāyānyeṣu kumbheṣu kim-artham-anudhāvanam ॥173॥

Tr. *śṛṅkhalā, jīvacāla* and *meru* are esoteric practices. Without them what is the use of practising other *kumbhakas*? 173.

योगदीक्षां विना कुर्वन् वातग्रन्थिं लभते ध्रुवम् ।
सर्वज्ञेन शिवेनोक्तं पूजां[3] सन्त्यज्य मामकीम् ॥
युज्यतः सततं देवि योगो नाशाय जायते ॥ १७४ ॥[4]
yoga-dīkṣāṃ vinā kurvan vāta-granthiṃ labhate dhruvam।
sarvajñena śivenoktaṃ pūjāṃ santyajya māmakīm ॥
yujyataḥ satataṃ devi yogo nāśāya jāyate ॥ 174 ॥

Tr. O *devi*! Without proper initiation into the practices, one is surely prone to get morbid vitiation of the vital air. According to *śiva*, without the devotion to *śiva*, if one undertakes the practice, it leads to harmful effects. 174.

Note. It has been maintained in the *haṭha-yogic* literature that erroneous practice of *prāṇāyāma* leads to vitiated *prāṇa* and causes diseases of *vāta*. In HP(K)-V.5 treatment of such diseases has been suggested. A specific mention has been made in the following verse of HP about *vāyu* or *prāṇa* going astray and not finding its way, it accumulates at one spot leading to several types of diseases. This condition of obstruction of *vāyu* in a particular spot is called *vāta-granthi:-*

"*pramādāt yogino vāyur-unmārgeṇa pravartitaḥ* ।
tadā mārgam anāsādya granthi-bhūtvā avatiṣṭhate ॥
tadā nānā-vidhā rogā jāyante vighna-kārakāḥ ॥

—By an error of the *yogī, vāyu* goes astray, (and) not finding its way (forward), accumulates at one spot. Then several types of diseases develop which create obstacles (in the path of *yoga*)." 174.

---

1. जीवचालश्चेति –J. 2. किमन्यं –HSC. 3. पूजा –J. 4. Verse not in A.

द्विविधा शृंखला प्रोक्ता स्वंगकुम्भान्तरादिका ॥ १७५ ॥

dvividhā śṛṅkhalā proktā svaṅga-kumbhāntarādikā ॥175॥

Tr. *śṛṅkhalā* is two-fold, one- *svaṅga-śṛṅkhalā* and the other *kumbhāntara-śṛṅkhalā*. 175.

असुः प्राणः[1] तदंगौ रेचपूरौ तदुक्तम्[2]—

asuḥ prāṇaḥ tad-aṅgau reca-pūrau tad-uktam—

Tr. *recaka* and *pūraka* are stated as the two aspects of *prāṇa-vāyu*--

पूरः[3] कुम्भः पुनः पूरः कुम्भपूरौ पुनः पुनः ।
पूरयेत् कुम्भकश्रान्तः[4] पूरश्रान्तश्च[5] कुम्भयेत् ॥ १७६ ॥

pūraḥ kumbhaḥ punaḥ pūraḥ
kumbha-pūrau punaḥ punaḥ ॥
pūrayet kumbhaka-śrāntaḥ
pūra-śrāntaś-ca kumbhayet ॥ 176 ॥

Tr. One should practise *kumbhaka* after *pūraka* again and again until one is exhausted. 176.

Note. There is great emphasis here on increasing the duration of *kumbhaka*. The more intense is the *kumbhaka*, more efficacious it becomes. Mild *kumbhaka* does not bring efficacious results. This is also the opinion expressed by *brahmānanda* while commenting on HP-II.49.

The line `*asuḥ prāṇaḥ*'—etc., seems to be incomplete as there is no quotation given as stated by the word `*taduktam*'. 176.

पूरकं पूरकं कुर्यात्तथा कुम्भं च कुम्भकम् ।
यावच्छक्तिस्ततः कुर्याद्रेचकं कुम्भकं पुनः ॥ १७७ ॥

pūrakaṃ pūrakaṃ kuryāt-
tathā kumbhaṃ ca kumbhakam ॥
yāvac-chaktis-tataḥ kuryād-
recakaṃ kumbhakaṃ punaḥ ॥ 177 ॥

---

1. प्राण –J. 2. Line not in A. 3. पुरः -J, परः -HSC. 4. कुम्भविश्रान्तः -HSC. 5. पूरविश्रान्त –HSC.

Tr. One should practise *pūraka* followed by *pūraka* again and again. Similarly, try to retain breath to the maximum capacity before exhalation. 177.

रेचकं कुम्भकं कुर्याद् गुरुदर्शितमार्गतः ।
रेचकं रेचकं कुर्यात् स्वंगशृंखलोदिता ॥ १७८ ॥
recakaṃ kumbhakaṃ kuryād guru-darśita-mārgataḥ ।
recakaṃ recakaṃ kuryāt svaṅga-śṛṅkhaloditā ॥ 178 ॥

Tr. In the same manner, one should exhale and hold the breath as instructed by a *guru*. The repeated attempt of *recaka* is known as *svaṅga-śṛṅkhalā*. 178.

हंसवेधं विना नैव कर्त्तव्यश्च कदाचन ।
ईश्वरप्रणिधानेन सिध्यते नात्र संशयः ॥ १७९ ॥[1]
haṃsa-vedhaṃ vinā naiva karttavyaś-ca kadācana ।
īśvara-praṇidhānena sidhyate nātra saṃśayaḥ ॥ 179 ॥

Tr. This should never be parctised without *haṃ sa-vedha*, which is, no doubt, attained through *īśvara-praṇidhāna* (devotion to God). 179.

Note. In this text, *haṃsa-vedha* has been referred to as a secret during the practice of *kumbhaka*. Although, the term *haṃsavedha* is not clearly defined, probably it refers to the condition of the working of *suṣumnā nāḍī*, during which this *kumbhaka*, called two-fold *śṛṅkhalā*, is prescribed.

The term *haṃsa-vedha* may be explained in the following manner. *ha* refers to *sūrya* or *piṅgalā nāḍī* and *sa* refers to *candra* or *iḍā nāḍī*, as has been stated in KP-113. *vedha* means to effect. Here *vedha* refers to effecting the working of both *iḍā* and *piṅgalā nāḍīs*, thus giving rise to the function of *suṣumnā nāḍī*. So, *haṃsavedha* maybe equated with the working of *suṣumnā nāḍī*.

Probably, the condition of *haṃsa-vedha* is attained through *īśvara-praṇidhāna*. 179.

1. Verse not in A.

गुरुमीशं समुल्लंघ्य यः कुर्यात् स विनश्यति ।
नाशिष्याय प्रदातव्यो नाभक्ताय कदाचन ॥
अपरीक्षितशिष्याय ददन्दुःखमवाप्नुयात् ॥ १८० ॥[1]

gurum-īśaṃ samullaṅghya yaḥ kuryāt sa vinaśyati ।
nāśiṣyāya pradātavyo nābhaktāya kadācana ॥
aparīkṣita-śiṣyāya dadan-duḥkham-avāpnuyāt ॥ 180 ॥

Tr. One comes to troubles without devotion to God and *guru*. This should not be divulged to any undevouted and unqualified disciple. Otherwise one faces misery. 180.

ब्रह्मरन्ध्रप्रवेशे[2] च कुण्डलीबोधनं[3] परम् ।
नाडीशुद्धिं मेरुसिद्धि[4]मारोग्यं च प्रयच्छति ॥
रेचकः क्षीणतां याति पूरकश्चातिवर्द्धते ॥ १८१ ॥

brahma-randhra-praveśe ca kuṇḍalī-bodhanaṃ param ।
nāḍī-śuddhiṃ meru-siddhim-ārogyaṃ ca prayacchati ॥
recakaḥ kṣīṇatāṃ yāti pūrakś-cātivardhate ॥ 181 ॥

यस्य नाथः स विख्यातो नमस्यः स सुरासुरैः ॥ १८२ ॥

yasya nāthaḥ sa vikhyāto namasyaḥ sa surāsuraiḥ ॥ 182॥

Tr. This practice leads to the attainment of purification of the *nāḍīs*, feeling of well-being, arousal of *kuṇḍalinī* and its entry into *brahmarandhra* and also success in *meru-kumbhaka*. Moreover, *recaka* becomes subtle and *pūraka* gets prolonged by the grace of the Lord who is adorned by the gods and the demons alike. 181-182.

कुम्भेऽन्य[5]कुम्भसंयोगात् स्यात् कुम्भान्तरशृंखला ।
विचित्रफलदा चेयं गुरुदर्शितमार्गतः ॥ १८३ ॥

kumbhe'nya-kumbha-saṃyogāt
syāt kumbhāntara-śṛṅkhalā ॥
vicitra-phaladā ceyaṃ
guru-darśita-mārgataḥ ॥ 183 ॥

---

1. Verse not in A. 2. ब्रह्मरन्ध्रप्रवेशं –HSC. 3. कुण्डल्योद्बोधनं –HSC. 4. मरुच्छुद्धिं –HSC. 5. कुम्भोन्य-HTK.

Tr. *kumbhaka* followed by *kumbhaka*, as instructed by a *guru*, is *kumbhāntara-śṛṅkgalā*, which leads to surprising results. 183.

बलात् कुम्भितवायोश्च[1] हृदयात् प्राणचालनम् ॥ १८४ ॥
balāt kumbhita-vāyoś-ca hṛdayāt prāṇa-cālanam ॥ 184 ॥
अधऊर्ध्वं स कुम्भस्तु जीवचालः शिवोदितः ।
विद्धानां सर्वसिद्धिः[2] स्यादविद्धानां तु ग्रन्थिदः ॥[3] १८५ ॥
adha-ūrdhvaṃ sa kumbhas-tu
jīva-cālaḥ śivoditaḥ ॥
viddhānāṃ sarva-siddhiḥ syād-
aviddhānāṃ tu granthidaḥ ॥ 185 ॥

Tr. One should activate the *prāṇa-vāyu* downwards and upwards which is held forcibly inside. This is *jīva-cāla-kumbhaka* narrated by *śiva*. When *prāṇa* penetrates (into *suṣumnā*), it leads to all accomplishment, if not, it leads to its morbid vitiation. 184-185.

मेरुसिद्धिं समाध्यन्तां[4] साधयेत् सिद्धिवृन्दकम् ॥ १८६ ॥[3]
meru-siddhiṃ samādhyantāṃ
sādhayet siddhi-vṛndakam ॥ 186 ॥

Tr. Success in *meru* and other *siddhis* is attained at the end of *samādhi*. 186.

मूलबन्धस्ततः पूरस्ततो जालन्धरस्ततः ।
कुम्भस्तत उड्डियानस्ततो रेच इति ह्ययम् ॥
षडंगकुम्भकः प्रोक्तः शम्भुना सर्वसिद्धिदः ॥[3] १८७ ॥
mūlabandhas-tataḥ pūras-tato jālandharas-tataḥ ।
kumbhas-tata uḍḍiyānas-tato reca iti hyayam ॥
ṣaḍaṅga-kumbhakaḥ proktaḥ
śambhunā sarva-siddhidaḥ ॥ 187 ॥

---

1. नामोश्चेद्ध –J. 2. सर्वसिद्धि-J. 3. Line not in A. 4. समाध्यन्ता-HSC.

Tr. The components of *ṣaḍaṅga-kumbhaka* stated by *śambhu* are *mūlabandha, pūraka, jālandhara-bandha, kumbhaka, uḍḍiyāna* and *recaka* which lead to success. 187.

Note. *ṣaḍaṅga-kumbhaka* is a typical term used in this text. It refers to six aspects of *prāṇāyāma*, in which three phases of *pūraka, kumbhaka* and *recaka* along with the application of three *bandhas*, namely, *mūla-bandha, uḍḍiyāna* and *jālandhara-bandha* are included. Thus the three phases of respiration and the three *bandhas* make six aspects of the *prāṇāyāma*. These are *ṣaḍaṅgas* (six essential components). *kumbhaka* being synonym of *prāṇāyāma*, the term used here is *ṣaḍaṅga-kumbhaka*. In other text, it is also known as *tribandha-kumbhaka*. 186-187.

सर्वत्र रेचकं कुर्याच्छनैरेव न वेगतः ।
अर्कतूलं यथा नैव स्पन्दते पवनेन तु ॥ १८८ ॥[1]

sarvatra recakaṃ kuryāc-chanair-eva na vegataḥ ।
arka-tūlaṃ yathā naiva spandate pavanena tu ॥ 188 ॥

Tr. *recaka* should always be performed slowly and not rapidly, so as not even to move a piece of cotton with the expired air. 188.

Note. In all the varieties of *prāṇāyāma (kumbhaka) recaka* or exhalation is always done slowly. This is emphasized in HP-II.49. Commenting on this verse, *brahmānanda* writes: -

"*pūraka* may be done slowly or quickly. Even if it is done quickly there is no harm. But *recaka* should be invariably performed slowly. Quick exhalation leads to loss of energy. This is also the opinion of several writers" (BPS-12.216).

An indication of slow *recaka* lies in reducing the force of the air to the minimum. When such force is reduced, even the tuft of cotton of a sun-plant does not move with the exhaled breath. 188.

पूरयेदर्कनाड्यासु कुम्भयित्वा यथाविधि ।
रेचयेच्चेन्दुनाड्यासु[2] कुम्भकः कमलाभिधः ॥ १८९ ॥

1. Verse not in A. 2. रेचयेचन्दुनाड्यासु –J, रेचयेच्चेदुभाभ्यांस –A.

pūrayed-arka-nāḍyāsu
kumbhayitvā yathāvidhi ||
recayec-ced-indu-nāḍyāsu
kumbhakaḥ kamalābhidhaḥ || 189 ||

Tr. When the air is inhaled through *sūrya-nāḍī* (right nostril) and exhaled through *candra-nāḍī* (left nostril) after systematically holding the breath, it is known as *kamala-kumbhaka.* 189.

Note. This technique resembles the technique of *sūryabheda* described earlier (KP-126), except the difference of producing sound while inhaling in *sūrya-bhedana.*

If the variant reading of A ms. is accepted, then one is supposed to exhale through both nostrils after inhaling through right followed by holding. 189.

पूरयेच्चन्द्रमार्गेण धारयित्वाध्वजायुधे ।
रेचयेत्तमुभाभ्यां चेत्कुमुदः कुम्भकः स्मृतः ॥ १९० ॥

pūrayec-candra-mārgeṇa
dhārayitvādhvajāyudhe ||
recayet-tam-ubhābhyāṃ cet-
kumudaḥ kumbhakaḥ smṛtaḥ || 190 ||

Tr. When the air is inhaled through the left nostril and after holding the breath, exhaled through both the nostrils, it is called *kumuda-kumbhaka.* 190.

सकृत्सूर्येण चापूर्य धार्य चन्द्रेण पूरयेत् ।
धारयेच्च प्रयत्नेन रेचयेत् क्रमतस्तथा ॥
नेत्रकुम्भ इति ख्यातः क्रमतो व्युत्क्रमादपि ॥ १९१ ॥

sakṛt-sūryeṇa cāpūrya dhārya candreṇa pūrayet |
dhārayec-ca prayatnena recayet kramatas-tathā ||
netra-kumbha iti khyātaḥ kramato vyutkramād-api || 191||

Tr. One should inhale once through *sūrya-nāḍī,* hold the breath and again inhale through *candra-nāḍī* and then after holding the breath exhale in the same order. This is known as *netra-kumbhaka.* This is done also in the reverse order. 191.

Note. The description of *netrakumbhaka* given here is called *krama-netra-kumbhaka.* As against this, when one inhales through *candra-nāḍī* (left nostril) and after retention (without exhaling), again inhales through *sūrya-nāḍī* (right nostril) and exhales through *candra-nāḍī* after retention, it becomes *vyutkrama-netra-kumbhaka*, which is also suggested as a practice. 191.

सकृच्चन्द्रेण चापूर्य धार्य सूर्येण पूरयेत् ।
नियम्य पूरयेन्नोभ्यां धारयित्वा यथाविधि[1] ॥
त्रिनेत्रकुम्भकः प्रोक्तस्त्रिनेत्रेण त्रिसिद्धिदः ॥ १९२ ॥[2]

sakṛc-candreṇa cāpūrya dhārya sūryeṇa pūrayet ।
niyamya pūrayen-nobhyāṃ dhārayitvā yathāvidhi ॥
trinetra-kumbhakaḥ proktas-tri-netreṇa
tri-siddhidaḥ ॥192॥

Tr. One should inhale once through the left and hold the breath, followed by inhalation by the right nostril and retain. Then again inhale the breath through both the nostrils, and hold the breath systematically (before exhalation). This is called *trinetra-kumbhaka* by *śiva*, which gives three-fold *siddhis.* 192.

घोणाभ्यां च मुखेनापि युगपत् पूरयेत् सदा ।
त्रिशूलिना त्रिशूलाख्यः कुम्भ उक्तस्त्रिशूलनुत् ॥ १९३ ॥[2]

ghoṇābhyāṃ ca mukhenāpi yugapat pūrayet sadā ।
triśūlinā triśūlākhyaḥ kumbha uktas-triśūlanut ॥ 193 ॥

Tr. One should always inhale through both the nostrils and mouth simultaneously and hold the breath (before exhalation). This is called *triśūla-kumbhaka* by *śiva* which removes three-fold sufferings. 193.

Note. Although the technique of exhalation in this *triśūla-kumbhaka* is not mentioned, probably it means exhalation through the nose and the mouth simultaneously after retention. 193.

---

1. यथाविधिः -J. 2. Verse not in A.

अमेरुमेरुभेदेन कुम्भं शम्भुर्द्विधावदत् ॥ १९४ ॥

ameru-merubhadena kumbhaṃ śambhurdvidhāvadat ॥194॥

Tr. According to *śambhu, meru* and *ameru* are the two types of *kumbhaka.* 194.

Note. Although the two aspects of *kumbhaka*, namely, *meru* and *ameru* have been referred to here, the description of *ameru* does not appear anywhere in the text. All the *kumbhakas* described in this text seem to fall in the category of *ameru-kumbhaka* (see note on KP-285-286). 194.

न वर्द्धयेन्निरोधं[1] च यथाशक्त्या सुसंयमम् ।
चरेत्स कुम्भकोऽमेरुश्चिरकालेन सिद्धिदः ॥ १९५ ॥

na vardhayen-nirodhaṃ ca yathā-śaktyā susaṃyamam ।
caret-sa kumbhako'meruś-cirakālena siddhidaḥ ॥ 195 ॥

Tr. When the breath-holding time is not increased and practised according to one's capacity, it is *ameru-kumbhaka*, which gives results in the long run, if practised judiciously. 195.

अमुमभ्यसतः[2] पुंसो नैसर्गिकमेरुसम्भूतिः ।
बहुभिः कालैर्भूयादगण्यपुण्यैर्परा सुमतेः ॥ १९६ ॥

amum-abhyasataḥ puṃso
naisargika-meru-sambhūtiḥ ॥
bahubhiḥ kālair-bhūyād-
agaṇya-puṇyair-parā sumateḥ ॥ 196 ॥

Tr. With the prolonged practice of this, one attains perfection of *meru* easily through a great fortune. 196.

तस्य त्रिभूमिकत्वं चिरकालाभ्यासतो भूयात् ।
द्वादशनैसर्गिकतो ह्यधिकश्चेद्दैवयोगेन[3] ॥ १९७ ॥

tasya tri-bhūmikatvaṃ cirakālābhyāsato bhūyāt ।
dvādaśa-naisargikato hyadhikaś-ced-daiva-yogena ।197।

1. नेरोधं –J. 2. अमुमभ्यसत –J. 3. ह्यधिकाश्रेद्देवयोगेन –J, ह्यधिकाश्चेद्देवयोगेन –HSC.

मात्राः[1] प्रथमभुवि स्याद्दत्तात्रेयो द्रवीभावे[2] ।
अस्याः[3] द्विगुणां कम्पां[4] त्रिगुणा[5]मुत्थापिकां योगी ॥ १९८ ॥

mātrāḥ prathama-bhuvi syād-dattātreyo dravībhāve ।
asyāḥ dviguṇāṃ kampāṃ triguṇām-utthāpikāṃ yogī ॥198॥

Tr. According to *dattātreya*, there are three stages of development with its prolonged practice. The first stage consists of twelve *mātrās* which may luckily increase. In this stage one gets perspiration. The second stage consists of twenty-four *mātrās* causing tremors and in the third stage with thirty-six *mātrās*, a *yogī* attains levitation. 197-198.

Note. *dattātreya* – an ancient authority of *yoga*. He was the son of *atri* and *anusūyā*. He is regarded as an incarnation of *viṣṇu*. He popularized the path of renunciation. Some of his famous disciples were *alakṣa, prahlāda, yadu* and *sahasrārjava*. The *yogic* texts contain the dialogues between *dattātreya* and these disciples.

There were many saints and traditions following *dattātreya* as their deity, such as *mahānubhāvas, dāsopanta, datta-sampradāya*. The name of *dattātreya* is associated with much published and unpublished literature, such as- *dattātreya yoga-śāstra, avadhūta-gītā, dattātreyopaniṣad, dattātreya-tantra, datta-gorakṣa-samvāda* etc. 198.

स्वेदे द्रवी भवेत् कम्प उत्थानेति तृतीयका[6] ।
आनन्दनिद्राघूर्णाश्च[7] रोमाञ्चध्वनिसंविदः ॥ १९९ ॥

svede dravī bhavet kampa utthāneti tṛtīyakā ।
ānanda-nidrā-ghūrṇāś-ca romāñca-dhvani-saṃvidaḥ ॥199॥

अंगमोटनकम्पाश्च भ्रमस्वेदप्रजल्पकाः ।
संविन्मूर्च्छादिकाश्चैव जायन्तेऽस्यां न संशयः ॥ २०० ॥

aṅga-moṭana-kampāś-ca
bhrama-sveda-prajalpakāḥ ॥
saṃvin-mūrcchādikāś-caiva
jāyante'syāṃ na saṃśayaḥ ॥ 200 ॥

---

1. मात्रा –HTK,HSC. 2. दत्तात्रेयोब्रवीत् द्रवीभावे –HTK, दत्तात्रेयो द्रवीभावे –HSC. 3. अस्या –HTK,HSC. 4. कम्पा –HSC. 5. त्रिगुणं –HTK,HSC. 6. कम्पे पोत्थाने तीतीयका-J. 7. घूर्माश्च-A,J.

Tr. In the third progressive stage, one experiences perspiration, ease, tremors, joy, trance, whirling, thrill, hearing of mystical sounds, bodily pain, sideward movements, inarticulate murmur and *samādhi.* 199-200.

पञ्चगुर्वक्षरैर्युक्तः[1] पलद्वयमितो हि यः ।
निसर्गतः कुम्भकोऽयं मतोर्द्धो[2] रेचकस्ततः ॥
अर्द्धपूरक इत्युक्तो मात्राकुम्भो[3] विशारदैः ॥ २०१ ॥

pañca-gurvakṣarair-yuktaḥ pala-dvaya-mito hi yaḥ ।
nisargataḥ kumbhako'yaṃ matordho recakas-tataḥ ॥
ardha-pūraka ityukto mātrākumbho viśāradaiḥ ॥ 201 ॥

Tr. When the breath is retained without force for a period of two *palas* (48 seconds) or time taken for recitation of five long vowels after inhaling for half the time (of recitation) and thereafter exhaling for the same period as of *pūraka*, it is called *mātrā-kumbhaka* by the learned. 201.

Note. The time ratio for inhalation, retention and exhalation in this *mātrā-kumbhaka* is 1: 2: 1, i.e., 24 secs : 48 secs : 24 secs. 201.

पञ्चविंशतिभिः प्रोक्तः पलैर्द्वादशमात्रिकः[4] ॥ २०२ ॥
pañca-viṃśatibhiḥ proktaḥ palair-dvādaśamātrikaḥ ॥202॥
पञ्चाशद्भिर्द्वितीयस्तु सपादघटिकोन्मितः[5] ।
तृतीय इति निर्दिष्टं दत्तात्रेयमतं मया ॥ २०३ ॥

pañcāśadbhir-dvitīyas-tu sapāda-ghaṭikonmitaḥ ।
tṛtīya iti nirdiṣṭaṃ dattātreya-mataṃ mayā ॥ 203 ॥

Tr. According to *dattātreya*, the first variety of *mātrā-kumbhaka* consists of twelve *mātrās* or twenty-five *palas* (of *kumbhaka*). The second variety consists of retention for fifty *palas* and the third one with one-and-a-quarter *ghaṭikās* (75 *palas*), (1 *pala*= 24 seconds). 202-203.

---

1. पञ्च गुर्व अरैर्युक्त-HSC. 2. निसर्गतः कुम्भकोयमथोध्वो –HSC. 3. मात्राकुम्भ-J, अर्धपूर(क)इत्युक्तो मात्राकुम्भो–HSC. 4. फलैर्द्वादिशमात्रिकः-HSC. 5. पञ्चाशुद्वितीयस्त सपादघटितोन्मितः -HSC.

नमः श्रीमन्महेशाय मेरुकुम्भोऽथ वक्ष्यते ।
मेरुकुम्भः शिवः साक्षान्नागुरुस्तमुपासते ॥ २०४ ॥[1]

namaḥ śrī-man-maheśāya meru-kumbho'tha vakṣyate ।
merukumbhaḥ śivaḥ sākṣān-nāgurus-tam-upāsate ॥204॥

Tr. After bowing down to Lord *maheśa (śiva), meru-kumbha* is now being described which is *śiva* Himself. This cannot be practised without a *guru.* 204.

बाह्याभ्यन्तरदेशेषु सञ्चारज्ञानतोऽथवा[2] ।
मात्रासंख्याश्वाससंख्या क्षणे यदवधारणे[3] ॥ २०५ ॥

bāhyābhyantara-deśeṣu sañcāra-jñānato'thavā ।
mātrāsaṃkhyā-śvāsasaṃkhyā kṣaṇe yad-avadhāraṇe ।205।

ईश्वरप्रणिधानेन[4] कुम्भको यत्र वर्द्धते[5] ।
एकमेरुर्मृडेनोक्तो[6] रहस्यं सर्वयोगिनाम् ॥ २०६ ॥

īśvara-parṇidhānena kumbhako yatra varddhate ।
ekamerur-mṛḍenokto rahasyaṃ sarva-yogināṃ ॥ 206 ॥

Tr. According to *mṛḍa (śiva),* when *kumbhaka* increases with the awareness of internal and external movement of *prāṇa* or determining the number of *mātrās* and respiration and devotion to God, it is called *eka-meru* which is the secret of all the *yogīs.* 205-206.

पूरकेनापि वृद्धेन द्विमेरुर्मेरुः च क्रमात्[7] ।
रेचकेनापि वृद्धेन त्रिमेरुः सिद्धिदायकः ॥ २०७ ॥

pūrakenāpi vṛddhena dvi-merur-meruḥ ca kramāt ।
recakenāpi vṛddhena tri-meruḥ siddhidāyakaḥ ॥ 207 ॥

Tr. With the increment in *pūraka* also it becomes *dvi-meru.* Similarly, with the increase of *recaka* it is *tri-meru.* When *meru* is practised progressively in this manner, it leads to success. 207.

1. Verse not in A. 2. बाह्याभ्यन्तरविषये सञ्चारज्ञानतो वा मन्दं –HTK. 3. मात्रासंख्या श्वासप्रमिति समयावधीरणतः-HTK. मात्रासंख्याश्चासमंस्याक्षणे यत्तावधारणैः -HSC. 4. मन्त्रस्य गणनैर्वापि –HSC,A. 5. मनुगणैर्वा क्रमशः प्रवर्धते यत्र वै कुम्भः -HTK. 6. एकमेरुर्मडेनोक्तो –HSC. 7. पूरकेणाभिबद्धेन द्विमेरुरोमेरुरोहणात –HTK, पूरकेनापि वृद्धेन द्विमेरो मेरुरोहणात –HSC,A.

षण्णिमेषो भवेत् प्राणः षड्भिः प्राणैः पलं स्मृतम् ।
पलैः षष्टिभिरेव स्याद् घटिकाकालसम्मिता ॥ २०८ ॥[1]

ṣaṇ-ṇimeṣo bhavet prāṇaḥ ṣaḍbhiḥ prāṇaiḥ palaṃ smṛtam।
palaiḥ ṣaṣṭibhir-eva syād ghaṭikā-kāla-sammitā ॥ 208 ॥

Tr. Six winkings make one *prāṇa* (respiration). Six *prāṇas* are equal to one *pala*. Sixty *palas* make one *ghaṭikā*. This is (an accepted) measure of time. 208.

तथा च पलप्रमाणं वार्त्तिके ॥[2]

tathā ca pala-pramāṇaṃ vārttike ॥

A measure of *pala* is also mentioned in *vārttika*.

रुद्रं शर्वं भर्गं स्थाणुं सोमं कन्दर्पघ्नं त्र्यक्षं पञ्चास्यम् ।
भीमं नागस्कन्धं भस्मांगं स्मृत्वा नत्वा कुम्भं कुम्भोवृद्धिम् ॥
शक्तेर्बोधं योगं सिद्धं सिद्धिं स सर्वमायुर्वृद्धिं प्राप्नोत्येवम् ।२०९।[1]

rudraṃ śarvaṃ bhargaṃ sthāṇuṃ somaṃ kandarpaghnaṃ tryakṣaṃ pañcāsyaṃ ।
bhīmaṃ nāga-skandhaṃ bhasmāṅgaṃ smṛtvā natvā kumbhaṃ kumbho-vṛddhim ॥
śaker-bodhaṃ yogaṃ siddhaṃ siddhiṃ sa sarvam-āyur-vṛddhiṃ prāpnotyevam ॥ 209 ॥

Tr. One should remember and bow down to *śiva* who is also called *rudra, śarva, bharga, sthāṇu, soma, kandarpaghna, tryakṣa, pañcāsya, bhīma, nāgaskandha, bhasmāṅga*. By this one attains increase in *kumbhaka*, arousal of *kuṇḍalinī*, longevity, all the *siddhis* and success in *yoga*. 209.

Note. The term *vārttika* refers to an explanatory note or a glossary. But which text is intended here is not clear. However, the term *pala* is equal to 24 seconds. (For other time measures see note on KP-158-163). 209.

डमरुं वालुकापूर्णं ताम्रपत्रं सरन्ध्रकम् ।
निधाय शैशिकद्वन्द्वे समधूच्छिष्टबन्धनात् ॥ २१० ॥

1. Verse not in A. 2. Line not in A.

ḍamaruṃ vālukā-pūrṇaṃ tāmra-patraṃ sarandhrakam ।
nidhāya śaiśika-dvandve samadhūcchiṣṭa-bandhanāt ।210।

प्रकल्प्य[1] गुरुदृष्टेन[2] यथा तन्मितकुम्भकम् ।
चरेत्सोऽयं घटीबन्धो[3] मेरुकुम्भकसाधकः ॥ २११ ॥

prakalpya guru-dṛṣṭena
yathā tan-mitakumbhakam ॥
caret-so'yaṃ ghaṭī-bandho
meru-kumbhaka-sādhakaḥ ॥ 211 ॥

Tr. One should tie up the joint of an hour-glass *(ḍamaru-yantra)* made of copper and fill it up with sand and make a hole at its bottom and use it for the measurement of time for *kumbhaka* as directed by the *guru*. This is called *ghaṭi-bandha*, which is used by the practitioner of *meru-kumbhaka*. 210-211.

Note: Hour-glass: an archaic hollow contraption filled with sand flow of which was used in the olden days to measure time. 210-211.

पूर्णः कर्षन् प्राणवायुस्त्वपानं
पादांगुष्ठान् मूलतो वापि नाभेः ।
आकण्ठं[4] हृत्खाद्वोत्प्रमातय्यं
पैतीत्युद्घातोऽयं योगिभिः सम्प्रदिष्टः[5] ॥ २१२ ॥

pūrṇaḥ karṣan prāṇa-vāyus-tvapānaṃ
pādāṅguṣṭhān mūlato vāpi nābheḥ ॥
ākaṇṭhaṃ hṛt-khād-vot-pramātayyaṃ-
paitītyudghāto'yaṃ yogibhiḥ sampradiṣṭaḥ ॥212॥

Tr. When one inhales *prāṇa* fully and draws the *apāna* from the toes, anus, navel, chest and takes it upto the throat, it is called *udghāta* by the *yogīs*. 212.

एकोद्घातो द्विरुद्घात[6]स्त्रिरुद्घातस्ततो मृदुः ।
मध्यमेरुस्तीव्रमेरुः[7] प्रत्याहारश्च धारणा ॥
ध्यानं समाधिरित्युक्तो मेरोः स्थूलभुवो दश ॥ २१३ ॥

---

1. प्रकल्प-HSC. 2. गुरुदष्टेन-HSC. 3. घटो बन्धो –HSC. 4. आकं –J. 5. आकण्ठहृत् वीद्वोत् प्रयातपय्यपैतीयुदघातोयं योगिभिः सम्प्रदिष्टः-A. 6. द्विरुद्घास-J. 7. मेरु-J.

ekodghāto dvir-udghātas-trir-udghātas-tato mṛduḥ ।
madhya-merus-tīvra-meruḥ pratyāhāraś-ca dhāraṇā ॥
dhyānaṃ samādhir-ityukto meroḥ sthūlabhuvo daśa ।213।

Tr. One *udghāta*, two *udghātas*, three *udghātas*, *mṛdu-meru*, *madhya-meru*, *tīvra-meru*, *pratyāhāra*, *dhāraṇā*, *dhyāna* and *samādhi* are stated to be the ten stages of *meru*. 213.

Note. The term *udghāta* occurs quite frequently in *purāṇas* and later *yogic* literature and has been given much diverse meanings that the word demands very careful consideration.

patañjali does not use the word *udghāta*. It is possibly introduced by *vyāsa* (on PYS-II.50) for the first time. *bālarāmodasīn* in his note on PYS-II.50 defines *udghāta* as the release of pressure exerted by the air trying to be exhaled and preventing exhalation. Physiologically, the upward pressure exerted by the inhaled air is called `the exhalatory pressure'. So long as a person is able to stand this pressure, retention of inhaled air continues and exhalation is prevented. Thus *udghāta*, according to *bālarāmodāsīn*, means exhalatory pressure felt at the end of *ābhyantara-kumbhaka* (internal retention of air).

According to comments of *bhoja* (PYS-II.50), the name *udghāta* is given to forceful contact of air with the palate. His definition of *udghāta* applies to *recaka* only, as he mentions—the air `that is driven from the root of the navel'.

The above two definitions represent a physiological phenomenon but do not relate to any time unit.

However, in VāPu-10:79-81, LPu-VIII.45-48, MPu and KūPu *udghāta* refers to twelve time units (*mātrās*) –"*udghātaḥ dvādaśa-mātrā smṛtaḥ*".

In all the *purāṇas udghāta* is equated with *prāṇāyāma* and is classified as *manda, madhya* and *uttama* or *tīvra* (i.e. mild, moderate and intense respectively).

Thus *udghāta* has been used in three senses, namely, i. exhalatory pressure, ii. forceful touch on the palate of the air being exhaled and iii. *kumbhaka.*

vyāsa uses six adjectives qualifying *udghāta.* They are, *prathama* (first), *dvitīya* (second) and *tṛtīya* (third) or *mṛdu*, *madhya* and *tīvra.*

The last three adjectives are the same that are used by the *purāṇas* for *kumbhaka*. Only the word *tīvra* is used instead of *uttama*. Here, *prathama* means *mṛdu*, *dvitīya* means *madhya* and *tṛtīya* means *tīvra*. Thus according to *vyāsa*, *udghāta* means *prāṇāyāma* which is further supported by the adjective `*saṅkhyā-paridṛṣṭaḥ*' (controlled through a set of ratio), which qualifies *prāṇāyāma*. (For elaborate discussion on *udghāta* see Yoga Mimamsa vol.VI.No.3, p.228-257).

The ten levels of *meru* are defined in quantitative time units along with the qualitative results. For example, if the latter stage is maintained twelve times of the units of the earlier stage, ultimately it leads to *samādhi*. We find similar view in SPu as well as in other *yogic* literature. 212-213.

प्रथमत्रितये[1] नाडीशोधनं वह्निदीपनम् ।
मृदौ स्वेदसमुद्भूतिर्मध्यमेरौ तु कम्पनम् ॥ २१४ ॥

prathama-tritaye nāḍī-
śodhanaṃ vahni-dīpanam ॥
mṛdau sveda-samud-bhūtir-
madhya-merau tu kampanam ॥ 214 ॥

तीव्रे खे[2] राजतेऽन्येषु स्वनामसदृशं फलम् ।
समाध्यन्तमिहोद्दिष्टं तत्तत्संज्ञा ततस्ततः ॥ २१५ ॥

tīvre khe rājate'nyeṣu
svanāma-sadṛśaṃ phalam ॥
samādhyantam-ihoddiṣṭaṃ
tat-tat-sañjñā tatas-tataḥ ॥ 215 ॥

Tr. First three stages lead to purification of the *nāḍīs* and increase of gastric fire. In *mṛdu-meru* perspiration is generated, in *madhya-meru* one experiences tremors and in *tīvṛameru* one levitates. In other stages upto *samādhi*, one gets the results as per the names indicate, such as *pratyāhāra*, *dhāraṇā*, *dhyāna* and *samādhi*. 214-215.

1. उद्घातत्रितये –HTK, HSC. 2. च-HSC.

Note. The symptomatic tests of *mṛdu* (mild), *madhya* (moderate) and *tīvra* (intense) *meru* have been given here. *mṛdu-meru* stage induces perspiration, *madhya-meru* stage brings about tremors and in the *tīvra-meru* the body is elevated. In HP(K)-II.12, the elevation of the body is substituted by the *vāyu* reaching *brahmarandhra*. *patañjali* has laid down the qualitative test for the progress in *prāṇāyāma* (PYS-II.50, 52-53). These may be summarized as follows:—

i. *kumbhaka* must become increasingly prolonged,

ii. it must become easier to practice,

iii. it must, step by step, decrease darkness obstructing illumination and,

iv. it must render the mind capable of deeper and deeper concentration.

patañjali does not mechanically look upon the progressive stages of *yoga* as a particular multiple of a particular preceding stage in duration, but clearly defines with qualitative tests by which each stage is to be judged. He has his own definitions of *pratyāhāra*, *dhāraṇā*, *dhyāna* and *samādhi*.

According to HTK-39:19, when *madhya-meru* is practised for two and a half *nāḍīs* (1 *nāḍī* = 24 minutes), it generates tremors in the body and remaining in *praṇava* for three *nimeṣas* (blinking), one experiences *tatva* (Reality) in the heart and in the state of *tīvra-meru*, when *nisarga-kuṃbhaka* arises, one levitates in *padmāsana*. If one sustains this state for three *ghaṭīs* (one *ghaṭī* =24 minutes) one certainly experiences loss of bodily consciousness (HTK-39:20). 214-215.

अथ प्रमाणमेतेषां रहस्यमपि कथ्यते ।
चतुरष्ट[1]द्वादशभिः क्रमादाद्याः पलैस्[2]त्रयः ॥ २१६ ॥

atha pramāṇam-eteṣāṃ rahasyam-api kathyate ।
catur-aṣṭa-dvādaśabhiḥ kramād-ādyāḥ palais-trayaḥ ।216।

ततः पञ्चदशोन्मानपलैरष्टादशोन्मितः[3] ।
परस्ततश्चतुर्विशपलैस्[4]तीव्र इहेरितः[5] ॥ २१७ ॥

---

1. चतुरष्टा-HSC. 2. फलैस्-HSC. 3. फलैः पञ्चदशो फलैरष्टादशोन्मितः-HSC. 4. फलैस्-HSC. 5. इहेरित-J.

tataḥ pañca-daśonmāna-palair-aṣṭādaśon-mitaḥ ।
paras-tataś-catur-viṃśa-palais-tīvra iheritaḥ ॥ 217 ॥

Tr. Their measures and secrets are being narrated further. The first three stages in sequence comprise of four *palas* (96 seconds), eight *palas* (192 seconds) and twelve *palas* (288 seconds). *mṛdu-meru* stage comprise of fifteen *palas* (360 seconds), *madhya-meru* of 18 *palas* (432 seconds) and *tīvra-meru* of 24 *palas* (576 seconds). 216-217.

निसर्गात्[1] द्वादशगुणः प्रत्याहारस्ततस्ततः[2] ।
स्वपूर्वा[3] द्वादशगुणाः[4] परे ज्ञेयाः शिवोदिताः ॥ २१८ ॥

nisargāt dvādaśa-guṇaḥ pratyāhāras-tatas-tataḥ ।
svapūrvā dvādaśa-guṇāḥ pare jñeyāḥ śivoditāḥ ॥ 218 ॥

Tr. According to *śiva*, the intensity of the stages from *pratyāhāra* onwards is twelve times more than the previous stage. Thus, twelve *prāṇāyāmas* make one *pratyāhāra*. Twelve *pratyāhāras* make one *dhāraṇā*. Twelve *dhāraṇās* make one *dhyāna* and twelve *dhyānas* make one *samādhi*. 218.

Note. Thus it will be observed that all the progressive stages of *yogic* development from *pratyāhāra* to *samādhi* are essentially linked with *prāṇāyāma*. 218.

अथ सूक्ष्मा इहोच्यन्ते मुनिवेदमिताः पराः ॥ २१९ ॥

atha sūkṣmā ihocyante muni-veda-mitāḥ parāḥ ॥ 219 ॥

Tr. Now the subtle *kumbhakas*, according to the *munis*, are being narrated. 219.

निसर्गसिद्धकुम्भाश्चेत्[5] प्रोक्तकालक्रमेण तु ।
वर्द्धते यत्र सा भूमिः[6] स्वस्वमानमिता भवेत् ॥ २२० ॥

nisarga-siddha-kumbhāś-cet prokta-kāla-krameṇa tu ।
vardhate yatra sā bhūmiḥ sva-sva-māna-mitā bhavet ।220।

---

1. निसर्ग -HSC. 2. प्रत्याहारस्ततः परम् -HSC. 3. स्वपूर्व -HSC. 4. द्वादशगुणः -J. 5. निसर्गसिद्धकुम्भा चेत् -J. 6. सासभूमिः-J.

Tr. When the duration of *kumbhakas* increases progressively as per the prescribed time units, one gets control over breath to one's capacity and gradually progresses towards the higher stages. 220.

Note. According to HTK-39:34 in *nisarga-siddha kumbhaka* when the *citta* gets merged in the *ādhāra (mūla)* and the stage of *sthānavāhā* measured by one breath arises through *prāṇāyāma*, one controls the *vāyus* like *kūrma, nāga* etc. in their respective places. 220.

शनैः शनैर्जितां भूमिमारोहेत यथा गृहम् ।
नोत्तरां भूमिमारोहेदजिताऽधरभूमिकः ॥
नो चेद् व्याध्यादयो विघ्ना भवन्त्यत्र न संशयः ॥ २२१ ॥

śanaiḥ śanair-jitāṃ bhūmim-āroheta yathā gṛham ।
nottarāṃ bhūmim-ārohed-ajitā'dhara-bhūmikaḥ ॥
*no ced vyādhyādayo vighnā bhavantyatra na saṃśayam*221

Tr. Just as one climbs the lower steps to reach the higher steps of a ladder in the house, similarly, one should progress slowly to the higher stages. If this is not followed, one has to face several troubles and diseases, in which there is no doubt. 221.

नाडीशुद्ध्युत्तरं मेरुस्थेषु विहरेत् सुखम् ॥ २२२ ॥

nāḍī-śuddhyuttaraṃ merustheṣu viharet sukham ॥ 222 ॥

Tr. Followed by the purification of the *nāḍīs*, one can comfortably undertake the practice of *meru-kumbhaka*. 222.

एकोन्मेषमिता स्पर्शा मूढा स्यात् षण्णिमेषिका ।
श्वासोन्मिता स्थानवाहा द्विश्वासा धातुशोषणा ॥ २२३ ॥

ekonmeṣa-mitā sparśā mūḍhā syāt ṣaṇ-ṇimeṣikā ।
śvāsonmitā sthāna-vāhā dvi-śvāsā dhātu-śoṣaṇā ॥ 223 ॥

Tr. (1) *sparśā*-- lasting for a fraction of second (one *unmeṣa*), (2) *muḍhā*— the time taken for six twinklings of the eyes, (3) *sthāna-vāhā*— one respiration (4 seconds), (4) *dhātu-śoṣaṇā*— eight seconds (two breaths). 223.

Note. In the state of *prāṇagā* (which may be equated with *dhātu-śoṣaṇā* in this context) measured by two breaths i.e. *dvi-śvāsā*, all (bodily) airs and the bodily constituents are made stable and limbs replenished. Two breaths *(dvi-śvāsā)* merge in the *ādhāra-tatva* (*pṛthvī* element). In *siddha-kumbhaka* one remains in *ādhāra-tatva* (*pṛthvī* element) for six *nāḍīs* (approximately 2 and a half hours) in a natural way (HTK-39:35). 223.

द्विगुणास्याः पुष्टिदा स्यात् पलमाना जितासना ।
अनाहता द्विपलिका चतुर्भिः स्याच्छुभाशुभा ॥ २२४ ॥

dviguṇāsyāḥ puṣṭidā syāt palamānā jitāśanā ।
anāhatā dvi-palikā caturbhiḥ syāc-chubhāśubhā ॥ 224 ॥

Tr. (5) *puṣṭidā*— 16 seconds, (6) *jitāsana*—one *pala* (24 seconds), (7) *anāhatā*— 2 *palas* (48 seconds), (8) *śubhāśubhā*— 4 *palas* (96 seconds). 224.

Note. The duration of *puṣṭidā* stage is given as four *śvāsas* i.e. equal to 16 seconds, by HTK. Here the duration is given double that of *dhātu-śoṣaṇā*. Thus, the duration of *dhātu-śoṣaṇā* comes to two *śvāsas* meaning eight seconds.

In addition, HTK-39:36 maintains that in the stage of *puṣṭidā*, when *citta* merges in *mūlādhāra*, all the *vāyus* enter into fourth *kumbhaka*. When *kumbhaka* is naturally held for six *nāḍīs* (2 and half hours), it nourishes the body.

Moreover, in the *jitāsanā* state, which is dominated by earth (element), one merges his *citta* in *ādhāra* for a *pala*. In an auspicious *āsana* while perfecting natural *kumbhaka* for six *ghaṭikās* (one *ghaṭikā* =24 minutes), one does not suffer at heart (HTK-39-37).

In the *ārambha* state of *jitāsanā*, through the practice of *prāṇāyāma, apāna* is controlled, for piercing *ādhāra* and for awakening of *bhujaṅgī (kuṇḍalinī)*, one should follow the instructions of a *guru* (HTK-39:39).

In the state of *anāhatā, śakti* along with fire merges in the heart for two *palas*. If *nisarga-siddha-kumbhaka* is maintained for six *nāḍīs* (1 *nāḍī* =24 minutes) the *anāhata* sound is heard (HTK-39:38). 224.

पलाष्टका स्मरहरा तिथिमानैश्च मार्गदा ।
त्रिंशत्पलमिता शक्तिबोधिनी सर्वसिद्धिदा ॥ २२५ ॥

palāṣṭākā smara-harā tithi-mānaiś-ca mārgadā ।
triṃśat-pala-mitā śakti-bodhinī sarva-siddhidā ॥ 225 ॥

Tr. (9) *smaraharā*— 8 *palas*, (10) *mārgadā*— 15 *palas*, (11) *śakti-bodhinī*— 30 *palas*. 225.

Note. In the state of *smara-harā* when *kuṃbhaka* is retained for six *ghaṭis* and the mind is retained at the *mūlādhāra* even for one *pala*, then a *muni* controls *kāma* (desire) (HTK-39:49).

nisarga-siddha-kumbhaka is maintained for 7 *ghaṭis*, while in the stage of *smara-harā*, it is maintained for 8 *palas* and a *muni* attains lustre and strength (HTK-40:90).

In the state of *mārgadā*, a *yogī* retains the mind for 15 *palas* by opening the gate of *suṣumnā* through the *vāyus* and retains it for one *prahara*, which is the state of *nisarga-kuṃbhaka*. This is known as the state of *paricaya* when *śakticāla* is perfected (HTK-39:50).

In the beginning of the practice of *prāṇāyāma*, *prāṇa* moves in its abode in the heart and due to fickleness of *citta*, *prāṇa* becomes active. Due to fire applied like an arrow through proper technique makes *prāṇa* subtle which has a tendency to move downwards and moves it at the seat of *śakti (kuṇḍalinī)* in the state of *mārgadā* (HTK-39:61). 225.

घटिकैकमिता शक्तिचालनोन्नयना परा ।
चित्तकम्पा द्विघटिका तद्विघ्नाग्निस्फुलिंगदृक् ॥ २२६ ॥

ghaṭikaika-mitā śakti-cālanonnayanā parā ।
citta-kampā dvi-ghaṭikā tad-vighnāgni-sphuliṅga-dṛk 226

Tr. (12) *śakti-cālanā*— one *ghaṭikā* (24 minutes), (13) *citta-kampā*— 2 *ghaṭikās* (48 minutes). 226.

Note. As a result of *nisarga-kumbhaka* retained for two *ghaṭikās*, the state of *citta-kampā* occurs for 10 *ghaṭikās* which removes mental fickleness but generates bodily tremors (HTK-45:52). 226.

जितासना[1] याममिता ता द्विघ्ना ज्योतिष्मती[2] ।
मात्राप्रकाशा प्रहरैश्[3]चतुर्भिः परिकीर्त्तिता[4] ॥ २२७ ॥

jitāsanā yāmamitā tā dvighnā jyotiṣmatī ।
mātrā-prakāśā praharaiś-caturbhiḥ parikīrtitā ॥ 227 ॥

Tr. (14) *jitāsanā*— one *yāma* (3 hours), (15) *jyotiṣmatī*— 2 *yāmas* (6 hours), (16) *mātrā-prakāśā*— 4 *praharas* (12 hours). 227.

अहोरात्रमिता[5] गन्धवती द्विघ्ना रसप्रदा ।
अहोरात्रैस्त्रिभिः प्रोक्ता रूपग्रहण[6]कारिणी ॥ २२८ ॥

ahorātramitā gandhavatī dvighnā rasa-pradā ।
ahorātrais-tribhiḥ proktā rūpa-grahaṇa-kāriṇī ॥ 228 ॥

Tr. (17) *gandhavatī*— one day and night (24 hours), (18) *rasa-pradā*—2 days (48 hours), (19) *rūpa-grahaṇa-kāriṇī*— 3 days (72 hours). 228.

चतुर्भिः स्पर्शवतिका पञ्चभिः शब्दसुश्रुतिः ।
बुद्धिदा षडहोरात्रैः सप्तभिः श्रुतिबोधना ॥ २२९ ॥

caturbhiḥ sparśavatikā pañcabhiḥ śabda-suśrutiḥ ।
buddhidā ṣaḍ-ahorātraiḥ saptabhiḥ śrutibodhanā ॥ 229 ॥

Tr. (20) *sparśa-vatikā*— 4 days, (21) *śabda-suśruti*—5 days, (22) *buddhidā*—6 days, (23) *śruti-bodhanā*— 7 days. 229.

अहोरात्रैर्वसुमितैर्जाठराग्निजयाभिधा ।
नवभिर्वाक्सिद्धिदा स्याद्दशभिश्चित्रदर्शना ॥ २३० ॥

ahorātrair-vasumitair-jāṭharāgni-jayābhidhā ।
navabhir-vāk-siddhidā syād-daśabhiś-citra-darśanā ।230।

Tr. (24) *jayā*—8 days, (25) *vāksiddhidā*— 9 days, (26) *citradarśanā*— 10 days. 230.

---

1. जिताशना-J. 2. ज्योतिष्मती भवेत्-HTK. 3. प्रहारैश्-HTK. 4. चतुर्भिः प्रहरै स्मृता –HTK. 5. अहोरात्रमितायां-HTK. 6. रूपग्रहणं –HTK.

एकादशाहोरात्रैः स्याद् वेगवत्यतिवेगदा ।
रविसंख्यैरहोरात्रैः स्यान्मनोजवदायिनी ॥ २३१ ॥
ekādaśāhorātraiḥ syād vegavatyativegadā ।
ravi-saṃkhyair-ahorātraiḥ syān-manojava-dāyinī ॥231॥

Tr. (27) *vegavatī*— 11 days, (28) *manojava-dāyinī*— 12 days. 231.

त्रयोदशमितैर्भूयात् खेचरीव गतिप्रदा ।
चतुर्द्दशदिनारभ्य[1] द्व्यधिकैर्द्व्यधिकैर्द्दिनैः ॥ २३२ ॥
trayodaśamitair-bhūyāt khecarīva gati-pradā ।
caturdaśa-dinārabhya dvyadhikair-dvyadhikairddinaiḥ ।232।
अष्टाविंशतिपर्यन्तमणिमाद्याः सुसिद्धयः[2] ।
भवन्ति भूमयश्चापि तासां नामभिरंकिताः ॥ २३३ ॥
aṣṭāviṃśati-paryantam-aṇimādyāḥ susiddhayaḥ ।
bhavanti bhūmayaścāpi tāsāṃ nāmabhir-aṅkitāḥ ॥ 233 ॥

Tr. (29) *gati-pradā*— 13 days, (30) *aṇimā*— 14 days, (31) *laghimā*— 16 days, (32) *prāpti*—18, (33) *prākāmya*— 20 days, (34) *mahimā*- 22 days, (35) *īśitvaṃ*- 24 days, (36) *vaśitvaṃ*— 26 days, (37) *kāmāvasāyitā*— 28 days. 232-233.

Note. The eight *siddhis* of *aṇimā* etc. have been included as eight stages of progress towards *meru-siddhi*. 233.

प्राप्तं ब्रह्मपदं[3] मार्गे विघ्नराशिरयं महान् ।
ईशस्य प्रणिधानेन किं वा साध्यं[4] न भूतले ॥ २३४ ॥
prāptaṃ brahmapadaṃ mārge vighnarāśir-ayaṃ mahān ।
īśasya praṇidhānena kiṃ vā sādhyaṃ na bhūtale ॥ 234 ॥

Tr. Reaching *brahmapada* is the path full of obstacles. It is not possible to attain it without devotion to or grace of god. 234.

मासान्निवर्त्तिका[5]भून्नवभिर्भूमयी ततः ।
सार्द्धवर्षात्तोयमयी त्रिभिस्तेजोमयी भवेत् ॥ २३५ ॥

---

1. चतुर्द्दशादिनारभ्य-HTK. 2. अणिमाद्या ससिद्धयः-J. 3. ब्रह्मयं –J. 4. न किं नासाध्यं –HTK. 5. मासान्निर्विर्त्तका-J; मासान्निवर्त्तिका भूयान् -HTK.

māsān-nivartikābhūn-navabhir-bhūmayī tataḥ ।
sārdhavarṣāt-toyamayī tribhis-tejomayī bhavet ॥ 235 ॥

Tr. (38) *nivartikā*— 1 month, (39) *bhūmayī*— 9 months, (40) *toyamayī*— one and a half years, (41) *tejomayī*— 3 years. 235.

षड्भिवर्षैर्वायुमयी द्विघ्नैर्व्योममयी[1] भवेत् ।
चतुर्विंशतिवर्षैः स्यात् प्रधानजयदायिनी ॥ २३६ ॥

ṣaḍbhir-varṣair-vāyumayī dvighnair-vyomamayī bhavet।
caturviṃśati-varṣaiḥ syāt pradhāna-jayadāyinī ॥ 236 ॥

Tr. (42) *vāyumayī*— 6 years, (43) *vyomamayī*- 12 years, (44) *pradhāna-jaya-dāyinī*— 24 years. 236.

पूर्वा विवेकख्यातिश्च धर्ममेघस्ततः परम् ।
गुरूपदिष्टकालेन जीवन्मुक्तमनःस्थिता[2] ॥ २३७ ॥

pūrvā vivekakhyātiś-ca dharmameghas-tataḥ param ।
gurūpadiṣṭa-kālena jīvanmuktamanaḥ-sthitā ॥ 237 ॥

Tr. (45) *viveka-khyāti* stage is followed by (46) *dharma-megha* stage after the period as narrated by the *guru* in which a *yogī* remains like a *jīvanmukta*. 237.

Note. *vivekakhyāti* is a term used by *patañjali* in PYS-IV.28 which means perfect discrimination coupled with detachment which leads to *samādhi* called *dharmamegha*. This discrimination is intellectual in as much as one adheres to the Eternal and the Real as against the ephemeral and transient which constitutes the world. According to *patañjali, dharmamegha* is the result of *vivekakhyāti* (PYS-IV.29). In this state nothing else has any value for a *yogi*. *dharma-megha-samādhi* is prior to *asaṃprajñāta-samādhi*.

jīvanmukta is a person who leads a life of a realized soul unaffected by the diversities of life and enjoys the Blissful state. 237.

अत ऊर्ध्वं ब्रह्ममयी परमात्मप्रकाशभूः ।
एकैवाव्याहता[3] तिष्ठेन्नान्या भूमिरतः परम् ॥ २३८ ॥

1. विघ्नैम-J, द्विघ्नै 12व्योमिमयी –HTK. 2. जीवन्मुक्तिमनस्थिता-HTK. 3. एकेवा न्याहता-J.

ata ūrdhvaṃ brahmamayī paramātma-prakāśabhūḥ ।
ekaivāvyāhatā tiṣṭhen-nānyā bhūmir-ataḥ param ॥ 238 ॥

Tr. Hereafter the *yogī* attains the final stage called (47) *pramātma-prakāśabhū* which is replete with *brahma* in which he remains engrossed without experiencing any other stage. 238.

Note. After narrating the last stage called *paramātma-prakāśa-bhū*, the author enumerates all the stages of *meru* with the word `*sapta-veda*', which means 47. 238.

एतास्तु भूमयो मेरोः[1] सप्तवेदमिताः[2] (४७) स्फुटाः[3] ।
अगर्भस्य सगर्भेषु निरूपणं कृतं मया[4] ॥ २३९ ॥

etās-tu bhūmayo meroḥ saptavedamitāḥ(47) sphuṭāḥ ।
agarbhasya sagarbheṣu nirūpaṇaṃ kṛtam mayā ॥ 239 ॥

Tr. These are the 47 stages of *meru* enumerated clearly. I have discussed *agarbha* in the context of *sagarbha*. 239.

Note. See note on KP-121. 239.

एतासां भूमिकानां यत्फलमाह[5] सदाशिवः ।
श्रद्धोत्साहप्रवृत्यर्थं तथा किञ्चिन्निरूप्यते ॥ २४० ॥

etāsāṃ bhūmikānāṃ yat-phalam-āha sadāśivaḥ ।
śraddhotsāha-pravṛtyarthaṃ tathā kiñcin-nirūpyate ॥240॥

Tr. The results of these stages have been stated by *sadāśiva*, out of which some are being narrated to motivate the practitioner with faith and enthusiasm. 240.

स्पर्शायां चित्तलीनत्वं परतत्वे प्रवर्त्तते ।
पुनः पुनश्च व्युत्थानं मूढायां घर्मसम्भवः ॥ २४१ ॥[6]

sparśāyāṃ citta-līnatvaṃ
para-tatve pravarttate ॥

---

1. मेरो –J. 2. सप्तवदमिताः -J. 3. स्फुटा-J. 4. अगर्भस्य सगर्भस्य सगर्भेषु निरूपणं –J. 5. फलमा सदाशिवः-J.
6. निद्रामूर्च्छाथवाशान्तिर्जायते तत्र योगिनः ।
स्थानवाहां तु सम्प्राप्य स्वस्थानेषु वायवः ॥ --extra in A.

punaḥ punaś-ca vyutthānaṃ
mūḍhāyāṃ gharma-sambhavaḥ ॥ 241 ॥

Tr. In *sparśā* state the *citta* tends to absorb in *paratatva* but repeatedly gets distracted. In *mūḍhā*, perspiration is generated. 241.

कूर्मनामादिका धातुशोषणा या तु धातुगा ।
वधं कुर्वन्ति ते तेषां पुष्टिदा या ह पोषका ॥ २४२ ॥

kūrma-nāmādikā dhātu-śoṣaṇā yā tu dhātugā ।
vadhaṃ kurvanti te teṣāṃ puṣṭidā yā ha poṣakā ॥ 242 ॥

Tr. In the state named *dhātu-śoṣaṇā* the impurities present in the *nāḍīs* like *kūrma* etc. are removed. That (state) which nourishes is *puṣṭidā*. 242.

Note. After narrating the results of *mūḍhā*, it was expected that the author gives the results of the stages of *sthāna-vāhā* and *jitā* along with the results of *dhātu-śoṣaṇā* and *puṣṭidā*. Probably the verse describing the results of *sthāna-vāhā* and *jitā* is somehow missing. 242.

जितासना भूमिसंस्थो योगी पीठे न खिद्यते ।
निमेषश्वासयोश्चात्र पेलवत्वं हि जायते ॥ २४३ ॥

jitāsanā bhūmi-saṃstho yogī pīṭhe na khidyate ।
nimeṣa-śvāsayoś-cātra pelavatvaṃ hi jāyate ॥ 243 ॥

Tr. The *yogī* who is established in the *jitāsanā* state, does not feel tired in the *āsana* and his eye movement and respiration get suspended. 243.

अनाहतायां कर्णाभ्यां श्रूयतेऽनाहतध्वनिः ।
तत्राप्युदासीनदशा न किञ्चिदपि चिन्तयेत् ॥ २४४ ॥

anāhatāyāṃ karṇābhyāṃ śrūyate'nāhata-dhvaniḥ ।
tatrāpyudāsīna-daśā na kiñ-cid-api cintayet ॥ 244 ॥

Tr. In *anāhatā* state one hears mystical sounds called *anāhata-dhvani* in the ears. One should remain indifferent about it without thinking of anything else. 244.

शुभाशुभाभ्यां भूम्यां चाकस्माच्छब्दः शुभाशुभः ।
योगिनो नित्यत्वेव कर्णयोराह शंकरः ॥२४५ ॥[1]

śubhāśubhābhyāṃ bhūmyāṃ
cākasmāc-chabdaḥ śubhāśubhaḥ ॥
yogino nityatveva
karṇayor-āha śaṃkaraḥ ॥ 245 ॥

Tr. According to *śaṅkara*, in *śubhāśubhā* state, the *yogī* suddenly hears in his ears the auspicious and inauspicious sounds (words) continuously. 245.

ततः स्मरहरायां तु कामं जयति लीलया ।
सुन्दर्यालिंगितस्यापि कामस्तस्य न जायते ॥ २४६ ॥

tataḥ smara-harāyāṃ tu kāmaṃ jayati līlayā ।
sundaryāliṅgitasyāpi kāmas-tasya na jāyate ॥ 246 ॥

वशे तिष्ठति स वापि जयेत् कामेन योगिराट् ।
त्यजेत्तथाप्युदासीनस्तत् संसर्गं विवर्जयेत् ॥ २४७ ॥

vaśe tiṣṭhati sa vāpi jayet kāmena yogirāṭ ।
tyajet-tathāpyudāsīnas-tat saṃsargaṃ vivarjayet ॥ 247 ॥

Tr. *smaraharā* state brings easy control over the passion and one does not get affected by lust even being embraced by the beautiful women. Thus the *yogī* masters the passion and it remains under his control. However, he should avoid contact with women and remain detached. 246-247.

मार्गदायां सुषुम्णायाः द्वारमुद्घाट्य वायवः ।
सूचीवेधनवद् विध्वा मध्यमायां चरन्ति ते ॥ २४८ ॥

mārgadāyāṃ suṣumṇāyāḥ dvāram-udghāṭya vāyavaḥ ।
sūcīvedhana-vad viddhvā madhyamāyāṃ caranti te ।248।

Tr. In *mārgadā* state the *vāyus* open the door of *suṣumṇā* and move freely into it like piercing of a needle. 248.

---

1. Verse not in A.

Note. *suṣumnā* is considered as the most important *nāḍī* in *yogic* literature. The oldest reference to *suṣumnā* is to be found in ChU-8.6.6. It is said to have started from the heart. The text says – "There are one hundred and one *nāḍīs* of the heart. One of them passes onto the head. The soul passing out through it gets immortality." So according to the ChU, the origin of *suṣumnā* is in the heart. However, GŚ-16 places the root of *suṣusmnā* and all other *nāḍīs* in the *kanda* below the navel. ŚS-II.22-23 traces the origin of *suṣumnā* in *mūlādhāra*. SN-1 describes *suṣumnā* as rising from the center of *mūlādhāra* to head. In respect of the course of *suṣumnā* through *meru-daṇḍa* (spinal column), there is no difference of opinion. *suṣumnā* splits itself into two branches after emerging from the spinal column. One of the two branches goes straight to *sahasrāra* and *brahma-randhra*, and the other through the *bhrū-madhya* and *ājñā-cakra* to *brahma-randhra*. *yogīs* look upon *brahma-randhra* as the upper opening of *suṣumnā* through which the *yogī*'s soul passes out. Opening of *suṣumnā* in the head is called *brahma-randhra*, as is seen in HP(L)-III.4.

To sum up, we find that according to different traditions of *yoga*, *suṣumnā* starts from the heart or from the *kanda* below the navel or from *mūlādhāra*. It passes through *meru-danda*. When it bifurcates, one branch goes directly to *brahma-randhra* and the other to *brahma-randhra* via *ājñā-cakra*. *suṣumnā* is located in-between *iḍā* and *piṅgalā*. 248.

शक्तिबोधिनीकायां तु मूलाधारस्थितां पराम् ।
चित्तवातनिरोधेन जागर्त्तीत्याह धूर्जटिः ॥ २४९ ॥

śakti-bodhinīkāyāṃ tu mūlādhāra-sthitāṃ parām ।
citta-vāta-nirodhena jāgarttītyāha dhūrjaṭiḥ ॥ 249 ॥

Tr. According to *dhurjaṭi (śiva)*, in *śakti-bodhinī* state *parā (śakti)* situated in *mūlādhāra* is awakened by the control of mind and *prāṇa*. 249.

ऊर्ध्वं कुण्डलिनी शक्तिचालनोन्नयनोद्भवा[1] ।
याति पश्चिममार्गेण मनोवातनिरोधनात् ॥ २५० ॥

1. नोद्भवो –J.

ūrdhvaṃ kuṇḍalinī śakti-cālanonnayanodbhavā ।
yāti paścima-mārgeṇa manovāta-nirodhanāt ॥ 250 ॥

Tr. *kuṇḍalinī* rises upwards and travels in the posterior path by the practice of restraint of mind and *vāyu* through (the practice of) *śakti-cālanā*. 250.

Note. Literally, *paścima-mārga* means posterior path. From the point of view of *haṭha-yoga*, *paścima-mārga* means the path of *suṣumnā* (HP-I.59). Commenting on this, *jyotsnā* explains *paścima-mārga* as *suṣumnā-mārga*.

According to SSP-I.7, *kuṇḍalinī* is the sentient life-force which is an evolute of *sūkṣmā-śakti*. *kuṇḍalinī(-śakti)* has five qualities such as *pūrṇatā* (completeness), *pratibimbatā* (reflectiveness), *prabalatā* (mightiness), *proccalatā* (upward motion) and *pratyaṅmukhatā* (interiorization). 250.

चित्तकम्पां तु सम्प्राप्य चित्तमस्य प्रकम्पते ।
अभ्यसेच्छान्तये योगी धैर्याच्छ्वासनिरोधने ॥
आत्मैकतानतायुक्तं न किञ्चिदपि[1] चिन्तनम् ॥ २५१ ॥

citta-kampāṃ tu samprāpya cittam-asya prakampate ।
abhyasec-chāntaye yogī dhairyāc-chvāsa-nirodhane ॥
ātmaikatānatā-yuktaṃ na kiñcid-api cintanam ॥ 251 ॥

अग्निस्फुलिंगदृग्भूगस्तेजोबिन्दुं प्रपश्यति ।
हृदि स्फुलिंगवत्तेन निद्रानाशोऽस्य[2] जायते ॥ २५२ ॥

agni-sphuliṅga-dṛg-bhūgas-tejo-binduṃ prapaśyati ।
hṛdi sphuliṅgavat-tena nidrā-nāśo'sya jāyate ॥ 252 ॥

Tr. A *yogī* in *citta-kampā* steadily practises control of breath along with the mind for tranquility and attunement with *ātman*, without thinking of anything else. Moreover, he perceives with his eyes brilliant light like the spark of a fire. When he sees the spark of light in the heart, he overcomes sleep. 251-252.

---

1. किंदपि –J. 2. निद्राशो –J.

व्युत्थाने स्यादुदासीनस्तत्रापीशानुचिन्तया ।
जिताशना[1]यामाहारगूथमूत्राल्पता भवेत् ॥
लाघवं स्निग्धता देहे योगिनः स्याच्छिवोदितम्[2] ॥ २५३ ॥

vyutthāne syād-udāsīnas-tatrāpīśānucintayā ।
jitāśanāyām-āhāra-gūtha-mūtrālpatā bhavet ॥
lāghavaṃ snigdhatā dehe yoginaḥ syāc-chivoditam ॥253॥

Tr. In spite of disturbances, in the state of *jitāśanā*, one should remain indifferent and contemplate on *īśvara*. In this state, the food intake, urine and faeces are reduced and the body of the *yogī* becomes light and smooth as narrated by *śiva*. 253.

ज्योतिष्मतीमनुप्राप्तस्तं प्रयुज्या तु भानवम्[3] ।
ज्योतिर्भानुभिरादीप्तं व्युत्थाने तमसि स्थितिः[4] ॥ २५४ ॥

jyotiṣmatīm-anuprāptas-taṃ prayujyā tu bhānavam ।
jyotir-bhānubhir-ādīptaṃ vyutthāne tamasi sthitiḥ ॥254॥

तेन स्वतेजसा विश्वं प्रकाशयति चेच्छया[5] ।
सुप्तोत्थितो[6]ऽन्धकारेऽपि स्वदेहं भानुवत्स्थितम् ॥
पश्यतीत्याह[7] भगवान् विश्वनाथो जगद्गुरुः ॥ २५५ ॥

tena svatejasā viśvaṃ prakāśayati cecchayā ।
suptothito'ndhakāre'pi svadehaṃ bhānuvat-sthitam ॥
paśyatītyāha bhagavān viśva-nātho jagad-guruḥ ॥ 255 ॥

Tr. Similarly, in the *jyotiṣmatī*, one is able to overcome ignorance and gains the knowledge of Reality as if one is awakened from the slumber, just as the brilliant light of the sun dispels the darkness. This is stated by *viśvanātha* who is *jagad-guru*. 254-255.

मात्राप्रकाशगो भूयात्[8] स्वात्मतत्वप्रकाशतः ।
इन्द्रियज्ञानविस्तारं[9] क्षमः कर्त्तुं जगत्यपि ॥ २५६ ॥

1.जितासना-HTK. 2. स्याच्चिरा दृढा-HTK. 3. ज्योतिष्मतीमनुप्राप्तसप्तज्यानुभानवं –HTK. 4. तमस्थितिः-HTK, तमसि स्थित –J. 5. स्वेच्छया-HTK. 6. सुप्तो स्थितो –HTK. 7. पश्यति साह-HTK. 8. भूयाः -HTK. 9. विस्तारे –HTK.

mātrā-prakāśago bhūyāt svātma-tatva-prakāśataḥ ।
indriya-jñāṇa-vistāraṃ kṣamaḥ karttuṃ jagatyapi ॥256॥

Tr. One gets enlightenment of one's *ātman* in *mātrā-prakāśā* and one is able to extend one's sensory abilities while remaining in the world. 256.

गन्धवत्यां दूरगन्धं[1] वेत्ति व्युत्थितचेतसि ।
रसप्रदा दूरसंस्थं रसं बोधयति क्षणात् ॥ २५७ ॥

gandhavatyāṃ dūra-gandhaṃ vetti vyutthita-cetasi ।
rasapradā dūra-saṃsthaṃ rasaṃ bodhayati kṣaṇāt ॥257॥

Tr. In the *gandhavatī* state one gets the extrasensory perception of smell. Similarly, in *rasapradā* one gets extrasensory perception of taste. 257.

रूपग्रहणकारिण्यां[2] दूररूपज्ञता भवेत् ।
स्पर्शवत्यां स्पर्शबोधो दूरतः सम्प्रवर्त्तते ॥
शब्दसुश्रुतिकायां[3] तु श्रूयन्ते दूरतो गिरः ॥ २५८ ॥

rūpa-grahaṇa-kāriṇyāṃ dūra-rūpajñatā bhavet ।
sparśavatyāṃ sparśabodho dūrataḥ sampravartate ॥
śabda-suṣrutikāyāṃ tu śrūyante dūrato giraḥ ॥ 258 ॥

Tr. The state of *rūpa-grahaṇa-kāriṇī* brings extrasensory perception of vision. In *sparśavatī* state a *yogī* gets extrasensory perception of touch.

In *śabda-suśrutikā* one gets the ability to hear the sounds from a remote source. 258.

पञ्चेन्द्रियज्ञानमिदं महत्स्वानुभवात्मकम् ॥
विश्ववर्त्तनमेतेन योगी वेत्त्यखिलं सुखात् ॥ २५९ ॥

pañcendriya-jñānam-idaṃ mahat-svānubhavātmakam ।
viśva-varttanam-etena yogī vettyakhilaṃ sukhāt ॥ 259 ॥

Tr. Thus are narrated the extrasensory perception of all the five senses based on rich personal experience. This helps a *yogī* easily gaining the entire knowledge of the functioning of the universe. 259.

1. दूरगन्ध –HTK. 2. सूर्यग्रहणकारिण्यां –J. 3. शब्दश्रुतिकायां –HTK.

बुद्धिदायां[1] महाबुद्धिर्योगिनः सम्प्रवर्त्तते ।
यया[2] विश्वं ज्ञानविश्वं वितर्क्या भाति यदृतम्[3] ॥ २६० ॥
buddhidāyāṃ mahā-buddhir-yoginaḥ sampravarttate ।
yayā viśvaṃ jñāna-viśvaṃ vitarkyā bhāti yad-ṛtam ।260।

Tr. In *buddhidā* state a *yogī* develops a great insight into the nature of the universe and gets the knowledge about it. 260.

श्रुतिबोधनभूम्यां[4] वेदविज्जायते मुनिः ।
आब्रह्मविश्ववेतृत्वं व्युत्थाने सम्प्रवर्त्तते ॥२६१ ॥
śruti-bodhana-bhūmyāṃ veda-vij-jāyate muniḥ ।
ā-brahma-viśva-vetṛtvaṃ vyutthāne sampravarttate ॥261॥

Tr. In the state of *śruti-bodhanā*, a *yogī* becomes adept in the *vedas.* In *vyutthāna* state one acquires the knowledge of the universe and *brahman.* 261.

जाठराग्निजयायां[5] तु सहजस्थोऽपि[6] योगिराट् ।
न रोगः[7] क्षुत्पिपासाद्यैर्न बाधामुपगच्छति ॥ २६२ ॥
jāṭharāgni-jayāyāṃ tu sahajastho'pi yogirāṭ ।
na rogaḥ kṣut-pipāsādyair-na bādhām-upagacchati ॥262॥

Tr. In the state of *jāṭharāgni-jayā,* the *yogī* remains in his natural state and is not affected by disease, hunger, thirst etc. 262.

वाक्सिद्धिदायां वाक्सिद्धिः शापानुग्रहणकारिणी ।
चित्रदर्शनभूम्यां सुगुप्तकार्याणि[8] पश्यति ॥
व्युत्थाने तु विचित्राणि तत्र चेतो न विन्यसेत् ॥ २६३ ॥
vāk-siddhi-dāyāṃ vāk-siddhiḥ śāpānugrahaṇa-kāriṇī ।
citra-darśana-bhūmyāṃ sugupta-kāryāṇi paśyati ॥
vyutthāne tu vicitrāṇi tatra ceto na vinyaset ॥ 263 ॥

---

1. बुद्धिदायाः-HTK. 2. यथा-J. 3. यद्वतं-HTK. 4. श्रुतिबोधनभूम्यं तु –HTK. 5. जठराग्निजयायाः -HTK. 6. सहस्थो य –HTK. 7. निरोगः-HTK. 8. तु गुप्तकार्याणि-HTK.

Tr. In the *vāk-siddhidā* state, one attains superhuman power of speech which gives the ability to curse or grace. In *citra-darśanā* one perceives many secret worldly events which are obstructions and should be ignored. 263.

वेगवत्यां तु मनसो वृत्या सह शरीरकम् ।
जवोदयाद्यातुमिच्छेदिति शंकरभाषितम्[1] ॥
स्यान्मनोजवदायिन्यां[2] विश्वभूमण्डलक्रमे ॥ २६४ ॥

vegavatyāṃ tu manaso vṛtyā saha śarīrakam ।
javodayād-yātum-icched-iti śaṅkara-bhāṣitam ॥
syān-manojava-dāyinyāṃ viśva-bhū-maṇḍala-krame ।264।

Tr. According to *śaṅkara*, in *vegavatī*, by mere will one can accelerate the speed of the body and mind. In the state of *mano-java-dāyinī*, one is able to move anywhere in the universe. 264.

Note. Here the author refers to the PYS-III.37—"*te samādhāvupasargāḥ vyutthāne siddhayaḥ*"— meaning that the *siddhis* (supernatural powers) although may indicate some progress by the *yogī*, are potential obstructions on the path of *samādhi*. The *siddhis* referred to here are well known eight-fold supernatural powers enumerated as – *aṇimā* (power of becoming as small as an atom), *laghimā* (assuming excessive lightness at will), *prāpti* (power of obtaining anything), *prākāmya* (irresistible will), *mahimā* (increasing size at will), *īśitva* (superiority, greatness), *vaśitva* (power to bring anything under control) and *kāmāvasāyitva* (suppression of passion or desire, stoicism). These bring results as indicated by their names. 264.

शक्तिरर्द्धनिमेषेण भूमितत्वस्य सिद्धितः ।
खेचर्यां खगति[3]र्भूयाच्चिन्तनादपि योगिनः ॥ २६५ ॥

śaktir-ardha-nimeṣeṇa bhūmi-tatvasya siddhitaḥ ।
khecaryāṃ khagatir-bhūyāc-cintanād-api yoginaḥ ॥265॥

1. जयोदयाद्याति दग्धं तूलवद्योगवह्निना –HTK. 2. स्यान्मनोजवदायिन्या-HTK.
3. च गतिर् -HTK.

Tr. The *khecarī* state brings power to a *yogī* through the control of earth element and the *yogī* at his will can move in the space in a fraction of a second. 265.

अणिमाद्यष्टभूमीनां[1] स्वनामसदृशं फलम् ।
समाध्युपसर्गाः[2] स्युर्व्युत्थाने सिद्धयस्त्विमाः ॥ २६६ ॥
aṇimādyaṣṭa-bhūmīnāṃ sva-nāma-sadṛśaṃ phalam ।
samādhyupasargāḥ syur-vyutthāne siddhayastvimāḥ । 266।

Tr. In the eight stages of *aṇimā* etc., one gets the results as suggested by the names. These are considered supernatural powers from the worldly point of view, but for *samādhi*, these are obstacles. 266.

निवर्त्तिकामनुप्राप्तो व्युत्थानैर्नोपहन्यते ।
यावद्विदेहकैवल्यं जीवन्मुक्तोऽयमीरितः ॥ २६७ ॥
nivarttikām-anuprāpto vyutthānair-nopahanyate ।
yāvad-videha-kaivalyaṃ jīvanmukto'yam-īritaḥ ॥ 267 ॥

Tr. After having attained the state of *nivartikā*, one is not affected by any obstructions. When *videha-kaivalya* state is attained, one is called *jīvanmukta*. 267.

Note. The meaning of *kaivalya* is detachment from the world, crossing of all the boundaries created by ignorance. In different scriptures, *kaivalya* has been termed differently as *mukti, mokṣa, apavarga, nirvāṇa* etc. According to the *upaniṣads*, there are two types of *kaivalya—jīvan-mukti* and *videha-mukti. jīvan-mukti* is a state in which a *yogi* performs his duties unattached with joy and sorrow. When the body of *jīvan-mukta* is destroyed in course of time, he attains *videha-mukti.* Here the author has equated *videha-kaivalya* with *jīvan-mukta* state. 267.

भूमय्यां[3] भूमिकायां तु श्रमणो वज्रसन्निभम् ।
देहं लभेद् भूमितत्वसिध्येत्युक्तं[4] कपर्द्दिना ॥ २६८ ॥

---

1. अणिमाद्यः अष्टसिद्धीनां –HTK. 2. समाधादुपसर्गाः -HTK. 3. भूमयां –J. 4. भूमितत्वं सिद्धत्युक्तं –HTK.

bhūmayyāṃ bhūmikāyāṃ tu
śramaṇo vajra-sannibham ॥
dehaṃ labhed bhūmi-tatva-
sidhyetyuktaṃ kaparddinā ॥ 268 ॥

Tr. According to *kapardī (śiva)*, in *bhūmayī* state, a *yogī* gets an adamantine body and attains control over earth element. 268.

तत्तत्त्वजयं[1] चैव शरीरमपि तन्मयम् ।
भूतस्वनामलिंगासु[2] भूमिष्वित्याह शंकरः ॥ २६९ ॥
tat-tat-tatva-jayaṃ caiva śarīram-api tanmayam ।
bhūta-svanāma-liṅgāsu bhūmiṣvityāha śaṅkaraḥ ॥ 269 ॥

Tr. According to *śaṅkara*, similarly, by controlling a *tatva* (element) the body gets influenced by that very *tatva*. 269.

प्राधानजयदायिन्यां प्रख्यादिगुणसाम्यताः[3] ।
यत्रास्त्यव्याकृताकाशे तद्वातरशनो[4] जयेत् ॥ २७० ॥
pradhāna-jaya-dāyinyāṃ prakhyādi-guṇa-sāmyatāḥ ।
yatrāstyavyākṛtākāśe tad-vāta-raśano jayet ॥ 270 ॥
करामलकवत्[5] पश्येद् ब्रह्माण्डमिह योगिराट् ।
काय[6]निर्माणमखिलं यथावत् पश्यति ध्रुवम् ॥ २७१ ॥
karāmalaka-vat paśyed brahmāṇḍam-iha yogirāṭ ।
kāya-nirmāṇam-akhilaṃ yathāvat paśyati dhruvam ॥271॥

Tr. In the state of *pradhānajayadāyinī*, a *yogī* gets the apperception of the balance of the three *guṇas*, like that of a clear sky. The *yogī* sees the whole universe like an Embolic Myrobalan (a fruit) at hand and is able to get the clear glimpse of evolution of the body. 270-271.

लिंगमात्रेण व्युत्थाने लिंगमात्रं[7] विशेषकान् ।
अविशेषांश्च[8] पुरुषमलिंगं च विलक्षणम्[9] ॥ २७२ ॥

1. तत्तत्वमयं–HTK. 2. भूतस्वर्नामलिंगासु–HTK. 3. प्रख्यादिगुणसाम्यया–HTK. 4. तद्वारशन–HTK. 5. करोमलकवत् -J. 6. काया-HTK. 7. लिंगमात्रे–HTK. 8. अविशेषश्च –HTK. 9. विलक्षणे–HTK.

liṅga-mātreṇa vyutthāne liṅga-mātraṃ viśeṣakān ।
aviśeṣāṃś-ca puruṣam-aliṅgaṃ ca vilakṣaṇam ॥ 272 ॥

वेत्ति पश्यत्यृतं[1] यावदित्युदासीनपूरुषः[2] ।
विवेकख्यातिदां येन तत्रोदासीनतामुतः ॥ २७३ ॥

vetti paśyatyṛtaṃ yāvad-ityudāsīna-pūruṣaḥ ।
viveka-khyātidāṃ yena tatrodāsīnatām-utaḥ ॥ 273 ॥

Tr. On the attainment of *vivekakhyāti* state, with the help of *liṅgamātra (mahat)*, an indifferent *yogī* gains the perception of the Reality *(ṛtaṃ)* through *viśeṣa* and *aviśeṣa*, *liṅga-mātra* and *aliṅga (viśeṣa*—five *mahābhūtas*, five *karmendriyas* and *manas*, *aviśeṣa*—five *tanmātrās*, and *ahaṅkāra*, *aliṅga*—*prakṛti)*, which leads to further indifference. 272-273.

Note. According to *sāṅkhya* philosophy, *puruṣa* principle, is in every way different from *puruṣa* as a person. *puruṣa* as principle does not involve *guṇas* as *prakṛti* does. *guṇas* have an objective reality. *puruṣa* principle is not objectively real which is said to be of the nature of *cetana* (pure consciousness). It is not a material cause of any effect.

The *puruṣa* who suffers, is a combination of *puruṣa* and *prakṛti*. By virtue of their *saṃyoga* with *puruṣa*, the *liṅga* appears as *cetana*. 272-273.

तत्परं रूपमाप्नोति धर्ममेघाह्वयं परम् ।
प्रत्ययान्तरमस्यात्र नोपपद्येन् महात्मनः ॥ २७४ ॥

tat-paraṃ rūpam-āpnoti dharma-meghāhvayaṃ param ।
pratyayāntaram-asyātra nopapadyen mahātmanaḥ ॥274॥

Tr. After this a *yogī* attains the state of *dharma-megha* in which there is no other experience. 274.

संस्कारबीजक्षयतः[3] क्लेशकर्मनिवृत्तये[4] ।
परमात्मप्रकाशाह्वां ततः प्राप्नोति भूमिकाम् ॥ २७५ ॥

saṃskāra-bīja-kṣayataḥ kleśa-karma-nivṛttaye ।
paramātma-prakāśāhvāṃ tataḥ prāpnoti bhūmikām ।275।

1. पश्यदृतं –HTK. 2. पूषः -J. 3. मू. अविशेषता अ यारीति -extra in J. 4. क्लेशकर्मनिवृये –J.

Tr. Thereafter, follows the state of *paramātma-prakāśā*, wherein a *yogī* burns the very seed of *saṃskāra*, which destroys the *karma* dominated by *kleśa*. 275.

Note. *kleśa-karma-nivṛtti* means complete removal of the past impressions of the actions influenced by five *kleśas*—namely—*avidyā, asmitā, rāga, dveṣa* and *abhiniveśa* (PYS-II.3). This takes place only after the attainment of `*dharma-megha-samādhi*' (PYS-IV.29).

saṃskāra-bīja means seed of past impressions which gives rise to the further *karmas.* Behavior and consciousness leave their effects behind and these determine subsequent behavior and consciousness. 275.

अगम्या वचसां शान्ता भूमिः संस्कारशेषतः ।
सा सीमा योगभूमीनां नित्यं तिष्ठन्ति योगिनः ॥ २७६ ॥

agamyā vacasāṃ śāntā bhūmiḥ saṃskāra-śeṣataḥ |
sā sīmā yoga-bhūmīnāṃ nityaṃ tiṣṭhanti yoginaḥ ||276||

Tr. This is the state of absolute peace, consisting of remaining *saṃskāras*, which is unintelligible and ineffable. This is the ultimate state of *yoga*, which should be maintained by a *yogī*. 276.

नास्य दृश्येन सम्बन्धो व्युत्थानेऽपि हि चिन्मयः[1] ।
लोकानां भासते देहे कर्माद्यस्य न किञ्चन ॥ २७७ ॥

nāsya dṛśyena sambandho vyutthāne'pi hi cin-mayaḥ |
lokānāṃ bhāsate dehe karmādyasya na kiñ-cana || 277 ||

Tr. Herein a *yogī* becomes *cin-maya* and does not get affected by coming into contact with the *guṇas*. Although he remains in the body, he is not influenced by *karma*. 277.

न देहमीक्षते देवो विरजं ब्रह्म चाग्रतः ।
विदेहोऽपीक्षते लोकैः सदेह इव चिन्मयः ॥ २७८ ॥

1. सदेहरद चिन्मयः -J.

na deham-īkṣate devo virajaṃ brahma cāgrataḥ ।
videho'pīkṣate lokaiḥ sadeha iva cinmayaḥ ॥ 278 ॥

Tr. Even the gods are not able to see his body before *brahma.* Even when he is without his physical body, he remains in his supreme spirit. 278.

सर्वाण्यस्य शरीराणि नैकमप्यस्य योगिनः ॥ २७९ ॥

sarvāṇyasya śarīrāṇi naikam-apyasya yoginaḥ ॥ 279 ॥

Tr. For such a *yogī* there could be several bodies and not just one. 279.

ब्रह्माविष्णवीशभवनाद्यनुयाति यथेच्छया[1] ।
मार्कण्डेयभुशुण्डादि सुखं भुक्तं न संशयः ॥ २८० ॥

brahmā-viṣṇvīśa-bhavanādyanuyāti yathecchayā ।
*mārkaṇḍeya-bhuśuṇḍādi sukhaṃ bhuktaṃ na saṃśayaḥ*280

Tr. He attains the abode of *brahmā, viṣṇu* and *īśa* according to the choice and undoubtedly enjoys pleasure like *mārkaṇḍeya, bhuśuṇḍa* etc. 280.

Note. *mārkaṇḍeya* was an ancient *ṛsi* who performed a great penance and obtained a long life. He was a devotee of *śiva* and was one of the exponents of *haṭha-yoga.* Some of the important texts on the name of *mārkaṇḍeya* are—*mārkaṇḍeya-smṛti, mārkaṇḍeya-purāṇa, mārkaṇḍeya-saṃhitā, mārkaṇḍeya-stotra.* 280.

फलान्युक्तानि भूमीनां यथा त्रिपुरान्तकः ।
चक्रेषु गुरुपूर्वस्य स्मरणेन प्रकाश्यते ॥ २८१ ॥

phalānyuktāni bhūmīnāṃ yathā tripurāntakaḥ ।
cakreṣu guru-pūrvasya smaraṇena prakāśyate ॥ 281 ॥

Tr. The results of these stages as have been narrated by *tripurāntaka (śiva),* are being described by the grace of ancient *gurus.* 281.

---

1. ब्रह्माविष्णवीशभवनान्यः तु याति निजेच्छया –J.

भूमिरापस्तथा तेजो वायुखं मन एव च ।
अन्ते परशिवश्चेति स स्मरेत् प्रथमं नगात् ॥ २८२ ॥

bhūmir-āpas-tathā tejo vāyu-khaṃ mana eva ca ।
ante paraśivaśceti sa smaret prathamaṃ nagāt ॥ 282 ॥

महद्रहस्यमत्रास्ति नाहं वक्तुं समुत्सहे[1] ॥ २८३ ॥[2]

mahad-rahasyam-atrāsti nāhaṃ vaktuṃ samutsahe ॥283॥

Tr. The five elements, namely, earth, water, fire, air and ether and mind and ultimately *paraśiva*—these seven principles should be contemplated upon. In this there is a great secret, which I am not able to disclose. 282-283.

शाम्भवीशिथिलाध्यानमुद्राभिरयमन्वितः ।
मेरुः शीघ्रं प्रसिध्येत रहस्यमिदमुत्तमम् ॥ २८४ ॥

śāmbhavī-śithilā-dhyāna-
mudrabhır-ayam-anvıtaḥ ॥
meruḥ śīghraṃ prasidhyeta
rahasyam-idam-uttamam ॥ 284 ॥

Tr. One attains success in *meru* when it is practised along with *śāmbhavī, śithilā-dhyāna* and *mudrā*. This is the secret. 284.

Note. The technique of *śāmbhavī-mudrā* described in HP(L)-VII.36 is : "Fixing up the mind on *antar-lakṣya* (an internal object) and keeping the eyes open without winking, is called *śāmbhavī-mudrā*". It is a *mudrā* in which concentration is attempted inside. This technique is suggested for the quick success in the practice of *meru*. 284.

अमेरुरपि कालेन स्वभ्यस्तोऽनेकजन्मभिः[3] ।
कस्मिंश्चित् सिध्यति[4] जन्तोः स्वतो[5] मेरुसमुद्भवात् ॥२८५॥

amerur-api kālena svabhyasto'neka-janmabhiḥ ।
kasmiṃś-cit sidhyati jantoḥ svato meru-samud-bhavāt ।285।

---

1. सत्सहे –J. 2. Line not in A. 3. स्वभ्यस्तेनेकजन्मनि –HSC. 4. सिध्यते –HSC. 5. स्वता –HSC.

Tr. With an efficient practice of *ameru* for several lives, one may succeed in attaining the stage of *meru* sometimes. 285.

सकला योगसिद्धिश्च मेरोरभ्यासतो[1] भवेत् ।
मेरुकुम्भं विना सिद्धिं य इच्छेत् स विमूढधीः ॥
वन्ध्यारतिः[2] पुत्राकांक्षी वन्ध्याशौ तावुभावपि ॥ २८६ ॥

sakalā yoga-siddhiś-ca meror-abhyāsato bhavet ।
meru-kumbhaṃ vinā siddhiṃ ya icchet sa vimūḍhadhīḥ॥
vandhyāratiḥ putrākāṅkṣī vandhyāśau tāvubhāvapi ।286।

Tr. All the supernatural powers in *yoga* are attained with the practice of *meru.* It will be unwise to expect the supernatural powers without the practice of *meru-kumbhaka*, like expecting a baby from a sterile woman. 286.

Note. The classification of *kumbhakas* is made into *ameru* and *meru* probably on the same lines as *sahita* and *kevala* state. Here also the goal is to reach *meru-kumbhaka* through *ameru-kumbhakas.* Thus it seems, *meru-kumbhaka* is a synonym for *kevala-kumbhaka.* In the *haṭha-yogic* literature we do not find elaborate and precise description of stages leading to *kevala-kumbhaka* as we find in this text. Moreover, various stages of progress are minutely described leading to the *meru-siddhi.* 285-286.

नैष योगः[3] प्रसिध्येत[4] विना ह्युत्तरसाधकम् ।
स चाप्तो हितकृन्मित्रं गम्भीरो[5] बुद्धिमान् सुखी ॥ २८७ ॥[6]

naiṣa yogaḥ prasidhyeta vinā hyuttara-sādhakam ।
sa cāpto hita-kṛn-mitraṃ gambhīro buddhimān sukhī ।287।

Tr. This *yoga* should not be divulged to anyone who is not an advanced practitioner. Such a *yogī* is a benefactor and friend. He is serious, wise and happy. 287.

अन्तःसमाधिस्थितयोगिराजे
हैयंगवीनैः सुरभीसमुत्थैः ॥

1. मेरोरभ्यातो –J. 2. बन्ध्यारतौ –HSC. 3. रोग-HSC. 4. प्रसिध्येते –HSC. 5. गभीरो –HSC. 6. Verse not in A.

सम्मर्द्दयेत् सोऽपि यथास्य चित्तं[1]
व्युत्थानमायाति तथा शिरोऽग्रम्[2] ॥ २८८ ॥[3]

antaḥ-samādhi-sthita-yogirāje
haiyaṅgavīnaiḥ surabhī-samutthaiḥ ॥
sammardayet so'pi yathāsya cittaṃ
vyutthānam-āyāti tathā śiro'gram ॥ 288 ॥

Tr. A *yogī* who is in deep *samādhi* should be applied massage with (cow) *ghee* on the head, so that he can regain consciousness. 288.

रहस्यमेतद् रघुवीरवाक्यामृतं निपीतकमुग्रदण्डम् ।
जित्वा पुरोक्तं विबुधाः खे न सुरा वा सुधियः प्रयान्तु ॥२८९॥[3]

rahasyam-etad raghuvīra-vākyāmṛtaṃ
nipītakam-ugra-daṇḍam ॥
jitvā puroktaṃ vibudhāḥ khe na
surā vā sudhiyaḥ prayāntu ॥ 289 ॥

Tr. This is the secret disclosed by *raghuvīra*, which may be taken in the form of nectar. Thus one overcomes (premature) death and enjoys heaven. 289.

Note. At the end of the text we find some stray verses referring to *agarbha* and *sagarbha-kumbhaka* as an appendage, where it is indicated that the text conforms to *agarbha kumbhaka paddhati* (see **Appendix-i**). It refers to *sagarbha-kumbhaka*, in which the technique of *kumbhaka* is accompanied by mental recitation of *mantra*, especially `*OM*', and meditation on it. The division of *agarbha* and *sagarbha-kumbhaka* is made on the basis of tradition. 289.

॥ इति श्रीमद्द्विजोदीच्यज्ञातिराजकुलाभिधात्
शिवरामात् समुद्भूतो रघुरामाभिधोऽकरोत् ॥

॥ iti śrīmad-dvijodīcya-jñāti-rāja-kulābhidhāt
śivarāmāt samudbhūto raghurāmābhidho'karot ॥

Thus ends the treatise by *raghurāma*, the son of *śivarāma* of the *udīcya* clan of the royal family.

***

1. शिरोत्थं –J. 2. यमास्यचित्तं –J. 3. Verse not in A.

Appendix—i

श्रीगणेशाय नमः ॥

ओमित्याख्ययाऽखिलश्रुतिष्वसकृत्सु गीतस्

तस्मै सगर्भवपुषे नम ईश्वराय ॥

यस्यान्तरा जगदिदं जगदन्तरायः

सृष्ट्यादिकृत् सकलपुरुषराजराजः ॥

हिरण्यगर्भो भगवान् सर्वसहाब्रवीत् ॥

शिवश्च ते वयं व्यक्तीकूर्मः कुम्भकमुत्तमम् ।

द्विविधः प्राणनियमः सगर्भागर्भभेदतः ॥

ध्यायनर्थ जपेन्मन्त्रं मनसा नियतानिलः ।

सगर्भः कुम्भकः प्रोक्तः पापहा पुण्यवर्धनः ॥

शतोन्मितोऽन्यतो मन्त्रसिद्धिदः शास्त्रभाषितः ।

अक्षरकमग्म वर्णाद्वर्ण चैवं पदात्पदम् ॥

तदर्थचिन्तनाभ्यासो मानसोऽत्र जपः स्मृतः ।

अगर्भः पुण्यपापाभ्यां रहितं प्रापयेत्पदम् ॥

शीघ्रं कुम्भकवृद्धिं च जप – ॥

Appendix –ii

Verses not found in *kumbhaka-paddhati* but cited in other texts as belonging to *kumbhaka-paddhati*

उभाभ्यां पूरयेद्वायुं कुम्भयित्वा यथाविधि ।
उभाभ्यां रेचयेद्वर्त्मगतिः कुम्भः शिवोदितः ॥ HTK-X.28
स्वमात्रैषा मध्यैषा षड्भिरीरितो जान्वोः ।
प्रदक्षिणकृतिर्नववरमसौ वरेति ॥ HTK
कान्तसप्तधाराप्रज्ञो जितश्वासाग्निहृत्तनुः ।
साक्षान् मधुमतीहस्य स्युरेताः सिद्धिभूमयः ॥ HTK-XLVII.33
आरूढयोगस्यैताः स्युर्व्युत्थाने सिद्धिभूमयः ।
सुसंयमपरिपाकाक्रमोत्तरशुभा मुनेः ॥ HTK-XLVI.50
सद्विवेकख्यात्यवधि स्यादौदासीनता ततः ।
परगं रूपगाप्नोति धर्गगेपाख्यं शुभम् ॥ HTK-XLVI.51

Appendix-iii

TABLE SHOWING THE DIFFERENT CHARACTERISTICS OF *TATTVAS* AND *SVARAS*

Name of element	Place	Shape	Quality	Colour	Taste	*bīja*	*svara*'s place	*svara*'s length (fingers)	Period (minutes)
Earth	*mūlādhāra*	square	smell	yellow	sweet	*laṃ*	middle of nostril	12	20
Water	*svādhiṣṭhāna*	half-moon	*rasa* chemical	white	astringent	*vaṃ*	lower part of nostril	16	16
Fire	*maṇipūra*	triangular	form	red	bitter	*raṃ*	upper part of nostril	4	12
Air	*anāhata*	hexagonal or round	touch	green or cloud color	sour	*yaṃ*	side of nostril	8	8
Ether	*viśuddha*	oval or sound dotted	sound	multi-farious	pungent	*haṃ*	rotating	20	4

Glossary

āma (155)—undigested content of food consumed which is toxic in nature giving rise to several diseases.

ameru-kumbhaka (194)—various types of *kumbhaka* leading to *meru-kumbhaka*.

anāhata (244)—fifth of progression towards *meru-kumbhaka*.

anāhata-dhvani (244)—internally aroused, unstuck mystical sound.

aṅga-moṭana (200)—a feeling of crushing pain in the body.

antaḥ-kumbhaka (28)—internal retention of breath during *prāṇāyāma*.

āntara-pūraka (24)—*pūraka* in which the inhaled air enters the opening of *suṣumnā*.

apāna (12)—an autonomic reflex activity downwards.

arka-nāḍī (189)—*sūrya-nāḍī, piṅgalā* or right nostril.

arka-vartman (164)—the passage of right nostril.

aviśeṣa (272)—the five *tanmātrās* namely, smell, touch, heat, taste and sound and *ahaṅkāra* (ego-consciousness).

bhū-mayī (285)—the thirty-seventh stage of *meru-kumbhaka* yielding an ability to have control over the earth element.

bhūta-śuddhi (157)—purification of the five elements namely earth, water, fire, air and ether.

bīja-mantra (113)—a single syllabled mystical letter with nasalized sound following a *mantra*.

brahma-randhra (181)—a point in the brain where *suṣumnā* reaches and is considered as the highest spot for concentration.

brahma-sthāna (156)—a synonym for *brahma-randhra*.

buddhidā (229)—twentieth stage of progress towards *meru-siddhi*.

candra-kumbhaka (41)—a synonym for *candra-bhedana.*

candra-vartman (165)—the passage of left nostril.

choṭikā-karaṇa (160)—snapping the fingers.

citra-darśanā (230)—the twenty-fourth stage towards the progress of *meru-siddhi.*

citta-kampā (226)—the eleventh stage in the progress of *meru-siddhi.*

daśa-vidha-prāṇa-nigraha (46)—control of five *prāṇa* namely, *prāṇa, apāna, samāna, vyāna* and *udāna* and five *upaprāṇas* namely, *nāga, kūrma, kṛkara, devadatta* and *dhanañjaya*, through the practice of *prāṇāyāma.*

devadatta (81)—control of *devadatta vāyu.* This is done by controlling yawning by closing the mouth.

dhanañjaya-jaya (213)—control of *dhanañjaya vāyu.*

dhāraṇā (213)—a state of concentration maintained for two hours on a single subject, which is considered twelve-times greater than the value of *pratyāhāra.*

dharma-megha (237)—the forty-fourth stage in the progress of *meru*; a name for *samādhi.*

dhātu-śoṣaṇā (223)—the third stage of progress on the path of *meru-siddhi.*

dhyāna (213)—an advanced stage of concentration (i.e. *dhāraṇā*), which is maintained for twenty four hours.

dṛśya (227)—that which is seen, a synonym for *prakṛti* consisting of three *guṇas.*

dvādaṣāṅgula (23)—twelve digits (nine inches).

dvi-meru (207)—when the time for *pūraka* is substantially increased it is so called.

eka-meru (207)—when retention of breath is increased with the help of *īśvara-praṇidhāna*, it is known as *eka-meru.*

gandhavatī (228)—the fifteenth stage of progress towards *meru-kumbhaka.*

gati-viccheda (15)—cessation of movement of inhalation—a synonym for *kumbhaka*.

gāyatrī (32)—a sacred *veda-mantra* composed in *gāyatrī* metre which consists of 24 letters as:

oṃ bhūr-bhuvaḥ svaḥ ı
tat-savitur-vareṇyaṃ bhargo devasya dhīmahi ı
dhiyo yo naḥ pracodayāt ıı

ghaṭikā-kāla (208)— a time unit for 24 minutes.

ghoṇā-yuga (157)—two nostrils.

ghūrṇa (199)—whirling of the body.

haṃsa-vedha (6)—the technique of controlling the activity of *iḍā* and *piṅgalā* and giving rise to the activity of *suṣumnā*.

iḍā (13)—the left nostril.

indu-nāḍī (189)—the left nostril.

īśvara-praṇidhāna (179)—devotion or act of devotion to God with detachment.

jālandhara (165)—one of the *bandhas* or neuromuscular locks in which the chin is put in the jugular notch by contracting the throat muscles. This is performed during *kumbhaka*.

jayā (230)—the twenty-second stage in the progression of *meru-siddhi*.

jitāsanā (227)—the twelfth stage in the progression of *meru-siddhi*.

jīva-cāla (184)—a type of *kumbhaka* in which the *prāṇa* is retained forcibly inside downwards and upwards.

jyotiṣmatī (227)—the thirteenth stage of progression of *meru-siddhi*.

kāka-cañcu (141,148)—beak of a crow.

kleśa-karma-nivṛtti (275)—annihilation of karma dominated by *kleśa*.

kleśa-karma-vipāka (1)—result of actions dominated by *kleśas*.

kumbhaka (20)—various techniques of holding the breath, a synonym for *prāṇāyāma*.

kumbha-mārga (8)—tradition of *prāṇāyāma*.

kumbhāntara-śṛṅkhalā (183)—intense practice of several subsequent *kumbhakas* in one breath.

kumbha-rāja (134)—a type of *kumbhaka*.

kuṇḍalī-bodhana (181)—awakening of the vital force called *kuṇḍalinī*.

kūrma-kumbhaka (79)—control of the winking reflex.

laghvakṣara (158)—a short vowel. The time taken for recitation of a short vowel is a measure of a *mātrā* (time unit).

liṅga-mātrā (272)—*mahat*—the first evolute of *prakṛti*.

madhyamā (248)—a synonym for *suṣumnā*.

madhya-meru (213)—fifth of the ten levels of *meru* in which one experiences tremors.

mahā-mātrā (163)—unit of time taken for recitation of '*a*' and '*ma*'.

manojava-dāyinī (231)—twentieth stage of the progression of *meru-siddhi*.

mano-mūrcchā (170)—enjoyable tranquility of mind.

mārgadā (225)—the eighth stage in the progression of *meru-siddhi*.

mātrā-kāla (158)—the measure of time.

mātrā-prakāśā (227)—the fourteenth stage on the progress of *meru-siddhi*.

meru (173)—final stage of *kumbhaka* which may be a synonym for *kevala-kumbhaka*.

meru-bhūmi (239)—forty-seventh progressive stage of *meru-kumbhaka*.

meru-siddhi (186)—success in *meru (kevala)* achieved at the end of *samādhi*.

mṛdu-meru (213)—fourth of the ten levels of *meru* wherein one experiences perspiration.

mṛga-kumbhaka (223)—a *kumbhaka* wherein *prāṇa* is held in the hip region.

mūḍhā (223)—the second stage in the progress of *meru-siddhi*.

mudrā (57)—internal neuromuscular lock leading to concentration.

mūla-bandha (186)—anal contraction, one of the six essential components of *meru*.

mūlādhāra (155)—one of the six important *cakras* located between anus and genital at the base of the spine.

nāda-śruti (49)—hearing of the unstuck mystical sound.

nāḍī-śuddhi (181)—purification of the *nāḍīs*.

niḥśvāsa (48)—exhalation.

nisarga-siddha-kumbhaka (220)— progressive development of *kumbhaka* as prescribed.

pala (208)—measure of time equal to twenty four seconds.

pañca-tatva (9)—five basic elements of earth, water, fire, air and ether.

parakāya-praveśa (55)—a process of entering into another body.

paramātma-prakāśa (238)—the forty-fifth stage in the progression of *meru-siddhi*.

paścima-mārga (250)—posterior path, the path of *suṣumnā*.

piṅgalā (13)—the right nostril.

prāṇa (11)—the upward activity in the body.

prāṇa-kumbhaka (17)—a synonym for *bāhya-kumbhaka*.

praṇava (17)—a synonym for '*om*'.

prāṇāyāma (5)—technique of retention of breath, a synonym for *kumbhaka*.

praśvāsa (10)—exhalation.

pratyāhāra (213)—one of the ten levels of *meru.*

pūraka (19)—inhalation.

puṣṭidā (224)—the fourth stage in the progress of *meru-siddhi.*

rasa-pradā (228)—the sixteenth stage in the progress of *meru-siddhi.*

recaka (19)—controlled exhalation.

śabda-suṣruti (229)—the nineteenth stage towards the progress of *meru.*

sahaja-kumbhaka (104)—effortless retention of breath all the time.

sahita-kumbhaka (86)—*kumbhaka* accompanied with inhalation and exhalation.

śakti-bodhinī (225)—the ninth stage in the progress of *meru-siddhi.*

samādhi (213)—the highest stage of contemplation, the tenth level of *meru.*

sama-kumbhaka (99)—a practice of suspension of breath irrespective of inhalation and exhalation.

samāna-kumbhaka (62)—holding of breath while concentrating on fire.

śāmbhavī (284)—vacant gaze in which the mind is concentrated on an internal object while keeping the eyes open without winking.

saṃskāra-bīja (275)—seed of the past impressions.

saṃskāra-śeṣa (276)—residue of the past impressions.

saṃvin-mūrcchā (200)—a synonym for *samādhi.*

śānta-kumbhaka (90)—a *kumbhaka* in which presence of *prāṇa* is visualized inside and outside.

sapta-dhātu (48)—the seven bodily constituents namely, chyle, blood, flesh, fat, bone, marrow and semen.

śiras (32)—the *veda-mantra* `*āpo jyoti raso'mṛtaṃ brahma-bhūr-bhuvaḥ svarom*' recited at the end of *gāyatrī-mantra*.

smara-harā (225)—the seventh stage in the progress to *meru-siddhi*.

sparṣā (223)—the first stage in the progress towards *meru-siddhi*.

sparṣa-vatikā (229)—the eighteenth stage in the progress of *meru-siddhi*.

śruti-bodhanā (229)—the twenty-first stage in the progress of *meru*.

śubhāśubhā (224)—the sixth stage towards the progress of *meru*.

śuddhi-kumbhaka (115)—a *kumbhaka* leading to purification of the *nāḍīs*.

suṣumnā (248)—the central path along the spine considered most important *nāḍī* in *yoga*.

svādhiṣṭhāna (155)—one of the six important *cakras* located in the genitals, commonly known as hypogastric plexux.

tāra (32)—a synonym for `*om*'.

tatva-jaya (269)—control of the five basic elements.

tejo-bindu (252)— perception of bright spot.

teho-mayī (235)—the thirty-ninth stage towards the progression of *meru*.

tīvra-meru (213)—one of the ten levels of *meru*.

toya-mayī (235)—the thirty-eighth stage in the progress of *meru*.

tri-meru (207)—a *kumbhaka* in which exhalation is prolonged.

ucchvāsa (48)—exhalation.

udāna-kumbhaka (68)—control of *udāna-vāyu*.

udghāta (9212)—exhalatory pressure, forceful touch of the air on the palate, *kumbhaka*.

vāk-siddhidā (23)—the twenty-third stage in the progress of *meru*.

vāta-granthi (174)—accumulation of *vāyu* at one spot due to obstruction in the passage.

vāyu-mayī (236)—the fortieth stage in the progress of *meru*.

vegavatī (231)—the twenty-fifth stage in the progress of *meru*.

viśeṣa (273)—the set of five *mahābhūtas*, five *karmendriyas* and *manas*.

viveka-khyāti (237, 273)—the discriminative knowledge, the forty-third stage in the progress of *meru*.

vyoma-mayī (236)—the forty-first stage in the progress of *meru*.

***

WORD INDEX

***

Alphabetical Index of Half-verses

प

फ

ब

भ

म

***

THE LONAVLA YOGA INSTITUTE (INDIA)

(Regd. No. 1439/1998/Pune)

A-7, Gulmohar Apartment, Bhangarwadi

Lonavla-410 401, Pune (India)

Tel: 0091-02114-270263 & 274431

Web: lonavalayoga.org

E-mail: lonayogalnl@vsnl.net

The Lonavla Yoga Institute (India) was founded in May 1996 by Dr. M. L. Gharote who was a student and collaborator of Swami Kuvalayananda, Founder of Kaivalyadhama Yoga Institute and a Pioneer of Scientific Yoga.

Activities of The Lonavla Yoga Institute (India)

1. To conduct or help conducting research in the field of pure and applied Yoga.
2. To edit or get edited text books on Yoga with notes and translations and publish them.
3. To prepare and publish catalogues, digests, indices or glossaries of Yogic texts and subjects allied to Yoga with a view to help critical studies of Yogic texts.
4. To publish Newsletter "Yoga Pradipa".
5. To organize seminars and conduct courses in Yoga and provide facilities for training individuals or groups of individuals in India or abroad.
6. To establish contacts and co-operate with the individuals and associations or organizations working in the field of Yoga in different aspects.
7. To give adequate guidance to the individuals and groups in the Yogic therapeutic matters.

Objectives

i. Publication of Yoga texts with translations in different languages.

ii. Catalogue of Yoga Manuscripts.

iii. Organization of Yoga Therapy Courses in different places with the help of affiliated or related Associations and Institutions.

iv. Organization of Yoga workshops for groups visiting India.

Publications

Within a short period of its existence the Institute has published the following books:

1. **Glossary of Yoga Texts**—Part-I & II—Dr. M. L. Gharote.
2. **Swami Kuvalayananda—A Pioneer of Scientific Yoga and Physical Education**—Dr. M. L. Gharote and Dr. M. M. Gharote.
3. **Yogic Techniques**—Dr. M. L. Gharote.
4. **Hatha Pradipika Vrtti by Bhojatmaja (Marathi)**—Ed. Dr. M. L. Gharote.
5. **Kumbhaka Paddhati or Science of Pranayama (second edition)**—Ed. Dr. M. L. Gharote & Parimal Devnath.
6. **Hathapradipika (10 chapters) with the Commentary Yogaprakasika by Balakrishna**—Ed. Dr. M. L. Gharote & Parimal Devnath.
7. **Yuktabhavadeva of Bhavadeva Mishra** (Original Sanskrit Text, English Summary and Critical Appraisal)—Ed. Dr. M. L. Gharote & Dr. V. K. Jha.
8. **An Introduction to Yuktabhavadeva of Bhavadeva Mishra** (English Summary and Critical Appraisal)—Ed. Dr. M. L. Gharote & Dr. V. K. Jha.
9. **Hatharatnavali** by Srinivasa—Critical edition, transliteration, translation, figures, notes and appendices.
10. **Pranayama- The Science of Breath**—Dr. M. L. Gharote.
11. **Siddhasiddhantapaddhati**—Dr. M. L. Gharote Dr. G. K. Pai.
12. **Encyclopaedia of Traditional Asanas**-- Dr. M. L. Gharote, et al.
13. **Posters of Yoga Practices** (Asanas & Kriyas.) In colour and black and white.

Future Publications

The Institute is working on the following texts and soon they will be published.

i. **Traditional Asanas and their Varieties** with illustrations and sequences.
ii. **Hathatattvakaumudi of Sundaradeva.**
iii. **Critical Edition of Yogopanishads.**
iv. **Concordance of Asanas and Pranayama.**
v. **Akulagama Tantra.**
vi. **Siddhanta-sekhara.**